TAB 4 U

A Concise Manual of Pharmacology

TAB 4 U
A Concise Manual of Pharmacology

Second Edition

Linto Antony A MBBS, DNB (Family Medicine)
Consultant Family Physician
Daya General Hospital, Valapad, Kunnamkulam
Thrissur, Kerala, India

Co-author

Femitha Rose Pharma D
Clinical Pharmacist
Daya General Hospital, Valapad, Kunnamkulam
Thrissur, Kerala, India

Foreword
MI Elsy

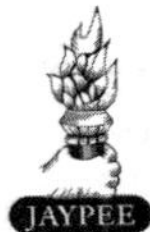

JAYPEE BROTHERS MEDICAL PUBLISHERS
The Health Sciences Publisher
New Delhi | London

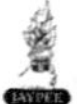 **Jaypee Brothers Medical Publishers (P) Ltd**

Headquarters

Jaypee Brothers Medical Publishers (P) Ltd
EMCA House
23/23-B, Ansari Road, Daryaganj
New Delhi - 110 002, India
Landline: +91-11-23272143, +91-11-23272703
+91-11-23282021, +91-11-23245672
Email: jaypee@jaypeebrothers.com

Corporate Office

Jaypee Brothers Medical Publishers (P) Ltd
4838/24, Ansari Road, Daryaganj
New Delhi 110 002, India
Phone: +91-11-43574357
Fax: +91-11-43574314
Email: jaypee@jaypeebrothers.com

Overseas Office

J.P. Medical Ltd
83 Victoria Street, London
SW1H 0HW (UK)
Phone: +44 20 3170 8910
Fax: +44 (0)20 3008 6180
Email: info@jpmedpub.com

Website: www.jaypeebrothers.com

Website: www.jaypeedigital.com

Inquiries for bulk sales may be solicited at: jaypee@jaypeebrothers.com

TAB 4 U: A Concise Manual of Pharmacology

First Edition: 2017

Second Edition: **2024**

ISBN: 978-93-5696-509-6

Printed in India at Sterling Graphics Pvt. Ltd.

Dedicated to

My Parents

Mr Antony AL

Mrs Karmala CD

Message

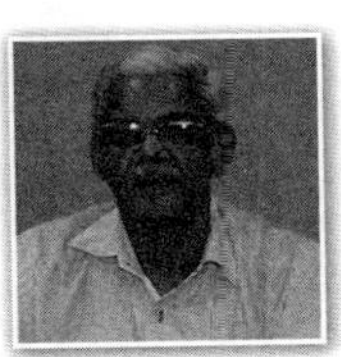

It is heartening to learn that the MBBS students of our institution have compiled all about the essentials of Pharmacology and are publishing the treatise entitled *Tab 4 U: A Concise Manual of Pharmacology*. The contents of the treatise reflect upon the classification, generic names, dosages, indications, side effects, contradictions and cautions for a vast majority of common medicinal drugs. For those who have the basic knowledge in Pharmacology, the *Tab 4 U* will serve as a ready reckoner, and the exam-going medical students of all parts of the country will be able to refresh their knowledge without strenuous exercise and lengthy hours of reading. It will also be a good guide for the general practitioners and specialists in Modern Medicine.

It will be another golden feather added to the crown of the Medicos of Jubilee Mission. I appreciate the pain-staking effort and academic enthusiasm of all the students who have toiled for materializing this work.

VK Ramankutty MD
Principal
Jubilee Mission Medical College and Research Institute
Thrissur, Kerala, India

Message

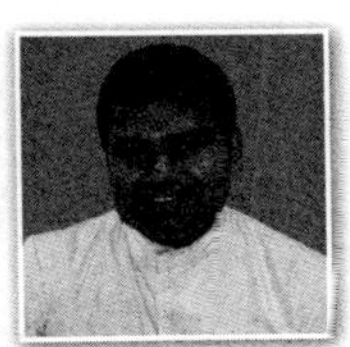

Proud to know that the MBBS students of Jubilee Mission Medical College and Research Institute, Thrissur, Kerala, India, are publishing *Tab 4 U: A Concise Manual of Pharmacology*, reflecting the classification, generic names, dosages, indications, side effects, contradictions and cautions for vast range of medicines. Lessening the burden of study, it surely will be a helping hand to all medical students of the country. Congratulations to the Jubilee Medicos efforts for a noble cause. Let similar initiatives help you and your colleagues in the future also to build-up the society.

Hearty congrats.

Fr Francis Pallikunnath
Director
Jubilee Mission Medical College and Research Institute
Thrissur, Kerala, India

Foreword

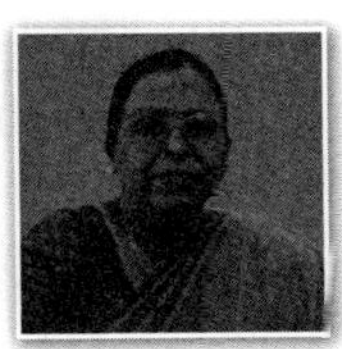

Medical education is now overloaded with too many subjects that the students find it very difficult to keep pace with all the information, especially, when they prepare for end-year examination. In this scenario, larger books do not find favor with students. Graduate students look for examination-oriented, easy-to-read, shorter textbook that covers the subject comprehensively, helping them to pass the examination without much effort.

It gives me immense pleasure to write a foreword for *Tab 4 U: A Concise Manual of Pharmacology*, a maiden effort of Linto Antony A and students of Jubilee Mission Medical College and Research Institute, Thrissur, Kerala, India. The book gives an overall idea about the drugs in pharmacology, their classifications, some important uses, adverse effects, etc. I am sure that the book will definitely serve the purpose of helping pharmacology students, especially during their study struggle on the previous days of university examination. However, the book is not a substitute for standard textbooks of pharmacology but will serve as quick reference.

I compliment the students wholeheartedly for their endeavor in bringing out the book and wish them all success.

MI Elsy MD
Professor and Head
Department of Pharmacology
Jubilee Mission Medical College and Research Institute
Thrissur, Kerala, India

Preface to the Second Edition

Admist the frenzy of torturous examination preparation, we often get lost ourselves. The monstrous textbook that has been our companion till then may not always give us a solution.

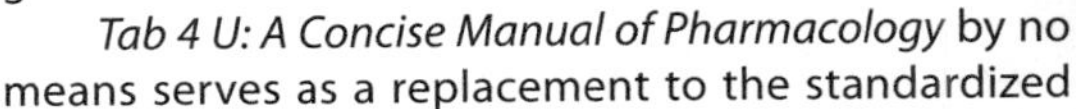

Tab 4 U: A Concise Manual of Pharmacology by no means serves as a replacement to the standardized textbooks but rather serves as quick-revision book. The book includes chapterwise classifications, mechanisms of action, uses, side effects, mnemonics and classification charts in the chapters. This book would definitely guide in the moment where time is short and a quick run thorough is required.

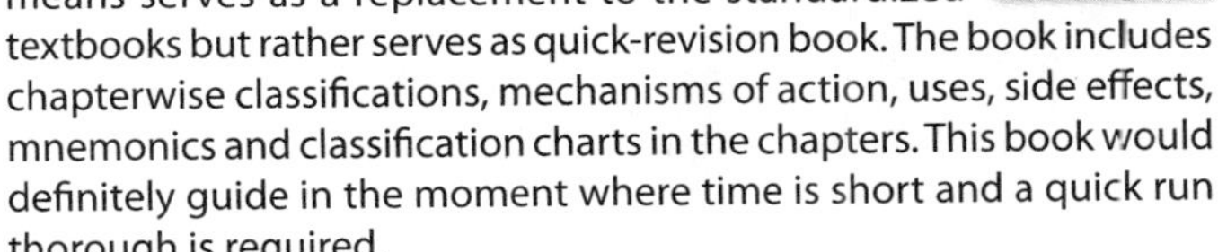

This venture would not have been possible without the everlasting support of my friends and I would be failing in my duty, if I do not gratefully acknowledge the contributions of Nidish Chandra and Don Davies. I also extend my heartfelt gratitude to my parents and teachers for their constant help, support and encouragement.

Linto Antony A

Preface to the First Edition

Admist the frenzy of torturous examination preparation, we often get lost ourselves. The monstrous textbook that has been our companion till then may not always give us a solution.

Tab 4 U: A Concise Manual of Pharmacology by no means serves as a replacement to the standardized textbooks but rather serves as quick-revision book. The book includes chapterwise classifications, mechanisms of action, uses, side effects, mnemonics and classification charts separately.

This venture would not have been possible without the everlasting support of my friends and I would be failing in my duty, if I do not gratefully acknowledge the contributions of Nidish Chandra and Don Davies. I also extend my heartfelt gratitude to my parents and teachers for their constant help, support and encouragement.

Linto Antony A

Acknowledgments

I heartily thank the following members for helping me in preparing the book in an elegant manner:

1. Kiran George (MBBS)
2. Nidheesh Chandra (MBBS)
3. Don Davis (MBBS)
4. Ajay Kuriyan (MBBS), Jubilee Mission Medical College and Research Institute, Thrissur, Kerala, India
5. Ajay Paul (MBBS), Jubilee Mission Medical College and Research Institute, Thrissur, Kerala, India
6. Ajmal Rahim (MBBS), Jubilee Mission Medical College and Research Institute, Thrissur, Kerala, India
7. Alwin Tony (MBBS), Jubilee Mission Medical College and Research Institute, Thrissur, Kerala, India
8. Frejin Francis V (MBBS), Jubilee Mission Medical College and Research Institute, Thrissur, Kerala, India
9. Jothsna Kuriakose (MBBS), Jubilee Mission Medical College and Research Institute, Thrissur, Kerala, India
10. Jugal James (MBBS), Jubilee Mission Medical College and Research Institute, Thrissur, Kerala, India
11. Kevin Joy (MBBS), Jubilee Mission Medical College and Research Institute, Thrissur, Kerala, India
12. Koshy T Sam (MBBS), Jubilee Mission Medical College and Research Institute, Thrissur, Kerala, India
13. Mariet Zachrias (MBBS), Jubilee Mission Medical College and Research Institute, Thrissur, Kerala, India
14. Manu Pradeep (MBBS), Jubilee Mission Medical College and Research Institute, Thrissur, Kerala, India

15. Nikil C John (MBBS), Jubilee Mission Medical College and Research Institute, Thrissur, Kerala, India
16. Praveen S (MBBS), Jubilee Mission Medical College and Research Institute, Thrissur, Kerala, India
17. Richie George (MBBS), Jubilee Mission Medical College and Research Institute, Thrissur, Kerala, India
18. Roshan Raju (MBBS), Jubilee Mission Medical College and Research Institute, Thrissur, Kerala, India
19. Vijay Krishnan (MBBS), Jubilee Mission Medical College and Research Institute, Thrissur, Kerala, India

Contents

Section 1: Drugs Acting on Central Nervous System

Section 2: Drugs Acting on Peripheral Nervous System

Section 3: Drugs Acting on Autonomic Nervous System

Section 4: Cardiovascular Drugs

Section 5: Respiratory System Drugs

Section 6: Gastrointestinal Drugs

Section 7: Drugs Acting on Kidney

Section 8: Autacoids and Related Drugs

Section 9: Hormones and Related Drugs

Section 12: Chemotherapy

Section 13: Miscellaneous Drugs

Abbreviations

A/C	:	Acute
A/E	:	Adverse Effect
ACE	:	Angiotensin Converting Enzyme
AMI	:	Acute Myocardial Infarction
AP	:	Action Potential
ARB	:	Angiotensin Receptor Blocker
AT	:	Angiotensin
BBT	:	Barbiturates
BP	:	Blood Pressure
BZD	:	Benzodiazepines
C/C	:	Chronic
C/I	:	Contraindication
C/S	:	Classification
CG	:	Cardiac Glycoside
CHF	:	Congestive Heart Failure
D/I	:	Drug Interaction
DN	:	Diabetic Nephropathy
DOC	:	Drug of Choice
FOC	:	Force of Contraction
GA	:	General Anaesthesia
GTN	:	Glycerine Trinitrate
HR	:	Heart Rate
LVF	:	Left Ventricular Failure
MOA	:	Mechanism of Action
NMJ	:	Neuromuscular Junction
PVD	:	Peripheral Vascular Disease
RAS	:	Reticular Activating System

S/E	:	Side Effect
SLE	:	Systemic Lupus Erythematosus
TCAs	:	Tricyclic Antidepressants
TDM	:	Therapeutic Drug Monitoring
UMNL	:	Upper Motor Neuron Lesions
VT	:	Ventricular Tachycardia
VF	:	Ventricular Fibrillation

1 SECTION

Drugs Acting on Central Nervous System

- Sedatives and Hypnotics
- Antiepileptic Drugs
- General Anesthetics
- Antipsychotic Drugs
- Antidepressant Drugs
- Antianxiety and Antimanic Drugs
- Opioid Analgesics
- Antiparkinsonian Drugs
- Central Nervous System Stimulants and Cognition Enhancers

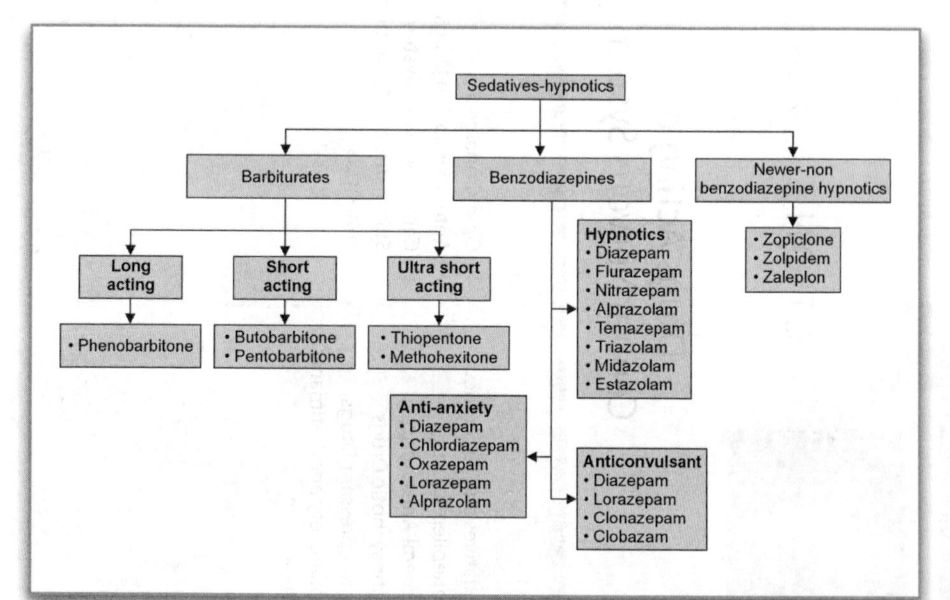
Sedatives-hypnotics
Barbiturates
Benzodiazepines
Newer-non benzodiazepine hypnotics
Long acting
Short acting
Ultra short acting
• Phenobarbitone
• Butobarbitone
• Pentobarbitone
• Thiopentone
• Methohexitone
Hypnotics
• Diazepam
• Flurazepam
• Nitrazepam
• Alprazolam
• Temazepam
• Triazolam
• Midazolam
• Estazolam
• Zopiclone
• Zolpidem
• Zaleplon
Anti-anxiety
• Diazepam
• Chlordiazepam
• Oxazepam
• Lorazepam
• Alprazolam
Anticonvulsant
• Diazepam
• Lorazepam
• Clonazepam
• Clobazam

CHAPTER 1

Sedatives and Hypnotics

CLASSIFICATION

1. BENZODIAZEPINES (BZD)

- Diazepam
- Lorazepam
- Midazolam
- Clonazepam
- Alprazolam

Site of action: Midbrain, RAS, Limbic system
Brainstem, Cerebellum

MOA: BZD bind to GABA receptor
↓
Increase frequency of chloride channel opening
↓
GABA facilitating action
↓
CNS depression

2. BARBITURATES (BBT)

Long acting	Phenobarbitone
Short acting	Butobarbitone
	Pentobarbitone
Ultrashort acting	Thiopentone
	Methohexitone
Site of action:	Mainly ascending RAS
MOA:	BBT bind to another site of GABA receptor ↓ Increase duration of chloride channel opening ↓ GABA mimetic and facilitating action ↓ CNS depression

3. NEWER NON-BZD

- Zopiclone
- Zolpidem

Benzodiazepines

Use of BZDs: **"A C" D I A** ze **P A M**
Alcohol withdrawal symptoms
Conscious sedation
Diagnostic and minor operating procedure

Insomnia
Anticonvulsant
Preanesthetic medication
Antianxiety
Muscle relaxant
A/E of BZDs:
- Floppy baby syndrome, if used in pregnancy confusion
- Blurred vision
- Tolerance
- Dependence

Barbiturates

Use of Barbiturates: **GoNADS**
General anesthesia
Neonatal jaundice of non-hemolytic type (enzyme inducing action)
Anticonvulsant action
Diagnostic aid in psychiatry
Sedation and hypnosis

A/E of BBTs: **RH DAM**
Rash
Hypersensitivity
Dependence and tolerance
Acute intermittent porphyria
Megaloblastic anemia

BZD antagonist: Flumazenil (used for BZD poisoning and reverse BZD anesthesia)

DOC for hypnosis in elderly—Zolpidem.

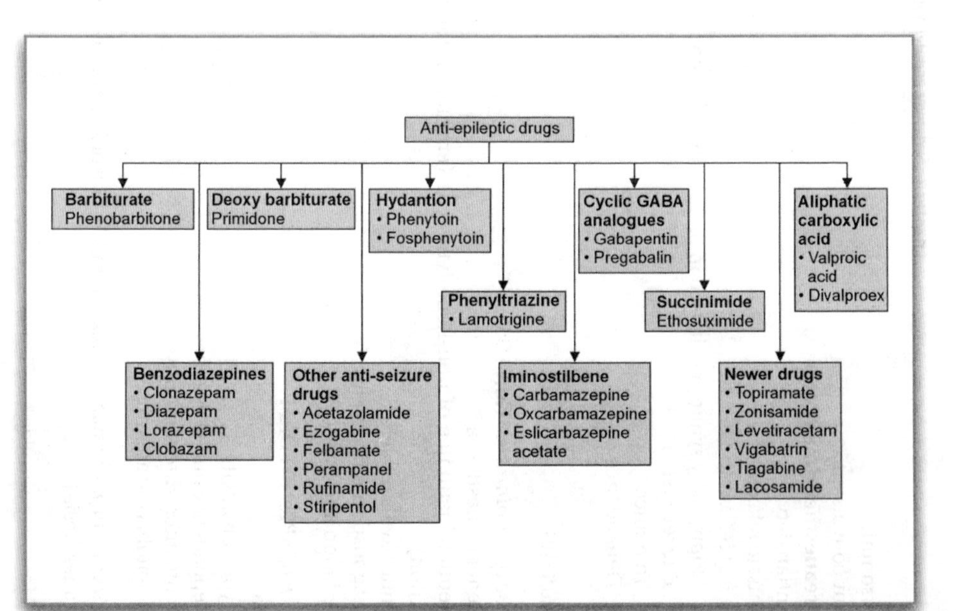
Anti-epileptic drugs
Barbiturate
Phenobarbitone
Deoxy barbiturate
Primidone
Hydantion
• Phenytoin
• Fosphenytoin
Phenyltriazine
• Lamotrigine
Cyclic GABA analogues
• Gabapentin
• Pregabalin
Succinimide
Ethosuximide
Aliphatic carboxylic acid
• Valproic acid
• Divalproex
Benzodiazepines
• Clonazepam
• Diazepam
• Lorazepam
• Clobazam
Other anti-seizure drugs
• Acetazolamide
• Ezogabine
• Felbamate
• Perampanel
• Rufinamide
• Stiripentol
Iminostilbene
• Carbamazepine
• Oxcarbamazepine
• Eslicarbazepine acetate
Newer drugs
• Topiramate
• Zonisamide
• Levetiracetam
• Vigabatrin
• Tiagabine
• Lacosamide

2 CHAPTER

Antiepileptic Drugs

CLASSIFICATION

SBI Big **C**onference **H**all

1. **S**uccinimide — Ethosuximide
2. **B**arbiturate — Phenobarbitone
3. **I**minostilbenes — Carbamazepine, oxcarbazepine
4. **B**enzodiazepine — Diazepam, lorazepam
5. **C**arboxylic acid — Valproic acid
6. **H**ydantoins — Phenytoin, fosphenytoin
7. **N**ewer agent — Topiramate, vigabatrin

MOA

a. 3, 6—Delay recovery of Na^+ channel from inactivated state
b. 2, 4—Facilitate GABA mediated chloride channel opening
c. I—It inhibits T type Ca^{2+} current in thalamic neurons
d. 5—a + b + c

Causes of Epilepsy

VITAMINS

Vascular events
Infection

Traumatic, toxins
Autoimmune
Metabolic, medication
Inborn error, induced by fever, hypoxia
Neoplasia
Shunt

PHENYTOIN

S/E:

PHENYTOIN
P-450 interactions
Hirsutism, **H**yperglycemia, **H**ypocalcemia
Enlarged gum (most common s/e)
precaution—maintain oral hygiene
Nystagmus
Yellow browning of skin
Teratogenicity—fetal hydantoin syndrome (Hypoplastic phalanges, cleft palate, harelip, microcephaly)
Osteomalacia
Interference with folate metabolism—Megaloblastic anemia
Neuropathies, vertigo, ataxia

Uses:

Generalized tonic—clonic seizure (5–8 mg/kg/day BD) in children, 100 mg BD, Max—400 mg/day in adult
Partial seizure
Trigeminal neuralgia
Status epilepticus

VALPROIC ACID

Uses: Absence, myoclonic, partial and generalized tonic—clonic seizures
Mania
Bipolar disorders

Dosage: 15–30 mg/kg/day

A/E: **VALPROATE**
Vomiting
Anorexia
Liver—hepatitis fulminant
Pancreatitis
Rashes
Orofacial and digital abnormality
Alopecia
Teratogenicity—spina bifida, neural tube defect
Elevation of liver enzyme

ETHOSUXIMIDE

- It only raises seizure threshold by acting on thalamocortical system.
- It selectively suppresses T current without affecting other type of Ca^{2+} or Na^{+} currents.
  Dosage: 20–30 mg/kg/day TDS

A/E:
- GI intolerance
- Tiredness
- Mood changes
- Agitation

DOC in absence seizures.

CARBAMAZEPINE

MOA:	Delays recovery of Na^+ channel from inactivated state It modifies maximal electroshock seizures as well as raises threshold to PTZ and electroshock convulsions
Uses:	Trigeminal and related neuralgias Manic depressive illness and acute mania
Dosage:	15–30 mg/kg/day Children, 200–400 mg TDS—adults
A/E:	Dose related neurotoxicity Hypersensitivity Increased incidence of minor fetal malformation Water retention and hyponatremia

DOC for GTCS, atonic, myoclonic seizures—valproic acid.
DOC for absence seizures—ethosuximide.
DOC for partial epilepsy—carbamazepine.
DOC for epilepsy in pregnancy—phenobarbitone.
DOC for febrile seizures—diazepam.
DOC for refractory convulsions—p araldehyde.

DIAZEPAM

Uses	– Status epilepticus – Tetanus – Eclampsia

Dose:	0.2–0.5 mg/kg slow IV. Max—up to 100 mg/kg Rectal instillation for febrile convulsions in children
S/E	Fall in BP Respiratory depression

DOC for emergency control of convulsions.

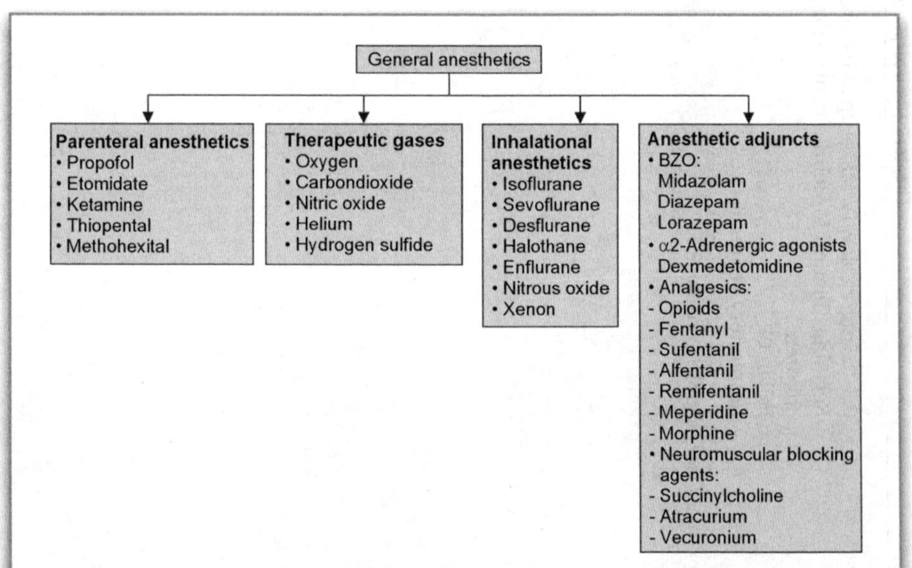

General anesthetics
Parenteral anesthetics
• Propofol
• Etomidate
• Ketamine
• Thiopental
• Methohexital
Therapeutic gases
• Oxygen
• Carbondioxide
• Nitric oxide
• Helium
• Hydrogen sulfide
Inhalational anesthetics
• Isoflurane
• Sevoflurane
• Desflurane
• Halothane
• Enflurane
• Nitrous oxide
• Xenon
Anesthetic adjuncts
• BZO:
Midazolam
Diazepam
Lorazepam
• α2-Adrenergic agonists
Dexmedetomidine
• Analgesics:
- Opioids
- Fentanyl
- Sufentanil
- Alfentanil
- Remifentanil
- Meperidine
- Morphine
• Neuromuscular blocking agents:
- Succinylcholine
- Atracurium
- Vecuronium

3 CHAPTER

General Anesthetics

1. INHALATIONAL

SHINE

Sevoflurane	*Use:* Good for pediatric Surgery *C/I:* Not used in closed circuit
Halothane	*Use:* In GA in asthmatics *S/E:* Malignant hyperthermia and hepatitis
Isoflurane	*Use:* In neurosurgery
Nitrous oxide	*Use:* Dental and obstetric surgery
Enflurane	

2. INTRAVENOUS

a. *Inducing agent:* **TEMP**

Thiopentone sodium
Etomidate

Methohexitone sodium
Propofol

b. *Slow Acting:* Benzodiazepines—diazepam, lorazepam, midazolam
Dissociative anesthesia—ketamine
Opioid analgesia—fentanyl

MOA: Potentiation of inhibitory neurotransmitter—BZD, propofol
Inhibition of excitatory neurotransmitter—N_2O, ketamine

Thiopentone Sodium

- Fast acting, redistribution present
- Used in control of convulsion and in narco analysis

S/E: Laryngospasm
Shivering and delirium
Precipitation of acute intermittent porphyria

Ketamine S/E

- Dissociative anesthesia
- Act on cortex and subcortical area
- Used in operation on head and neck, for burn dressing
- Good for hypovolemic patient

BP and HR
Intracranial pressure
Delirium-hallucination

KETAMINE

- **K**ids (Anesthetic in children)
- **E**mergence reaction (Hallucination)

- **T**halamocortical junction (site of action)
- **A**nalgesia
- **M**eals (can be given in full stomach)
- **I**ncrease all pressure (BP, IOP, ICT)
- **N**MDA antagonist excellent for asthmatic and hypovolemic patients.

HALOTHANE

- **H**yperthermia (malignant hyperthermia)
- **A**rrhythmia
- **L**iver toxicity
- **O**rthostatic hypotension
- **T**ocolytic
- **H**eart inhibition
- **A**sthma (used as general anesthetic in asthmatic)
- **N**on **E**xplosive

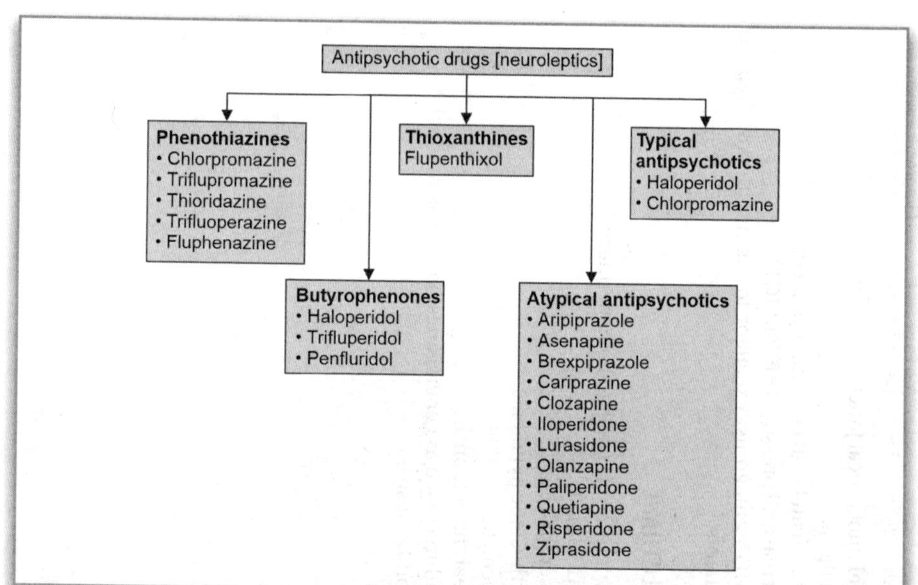
Antipsychotic drugs [neuroleptics]
Phenothiazines
• Chlorpromazine
• Triflupromazine
• Thioridazine
• Trifluoperazine
• Fluphenazine
Thioxanthines
Flupenthixol
Typical antipsychotics
• Haloperidol
• Chlorpromazine
Butyrophenones
• Haloperidol
• Trifluperidol
• Penfluridol
Atypical antipsychotics
• Aripiprazole
• Asenapine
• Brexpiprazole
• Cariprazine
• Clozapine
• Iloperidone
• Lurasidone
• Olanzapine
• Paliperidone
• Quetiapine
• Risperidone
• Ziprasidone

4 CHAPTER

Antipsychotic Drugs

CLASSIFICATION

♦ Phenothiazines	**TTC** **T**riflupromazine **T**rifluoperazine **C**hlorpromazine
♦ Thioxanthene's	Flupenthixol
♦ Butyrophenones	Haloperidol Trifluperidol
♦ Atypical Antipsychotics	**COR** **C**lozapine **O**lanzapine **R**isperidone

Uses: **SAMI**
Schizophrenia
As antiemetic—haloperidol
Mania
Intractable hiccups

MOA:

- Antipsychotic—mainly block dopamine receptors in mesolimbic and mesocortical area

- Atypical antipsychotics—block 5 HT_{2a} receptors in mesolimbic system

A/E:

Antipsychotics **PATAM**

Parkinsonism
Acute dystonia
Tardive dyskinesia
Add weight
Malignant neuroleptic syndrome

Atypical Antipsychotics

- Weight gain
- Hypotension
- Agranulocytosis—clozapine

DOC for treatment resistant schizophrenia—clozapine.
DOC for heat stroke, hiccups—chlorpromazine.
DOC for acute mania—haloperidol.

NEUROLEPTIC SYNDROME

- CPZ in normal individuals
- CAUSES—**PRE IPS**
- **P**aucity of thought
- **R**eduction in initiative
- **E**motional distress
- **I**ndifference to surroundings
- **P**sychomotor slowing
- **S**leep—tendency to go off but easily arousable

MALIGNANT NEUROLEPTIC SYNDROME

- High closes of potent antipsychotics
- Rigidity, tremor, immobility
- Fever, semiconsciousness
- HR and BP fluctuations
- Raised myoglobin
- Management—IV dantrolene

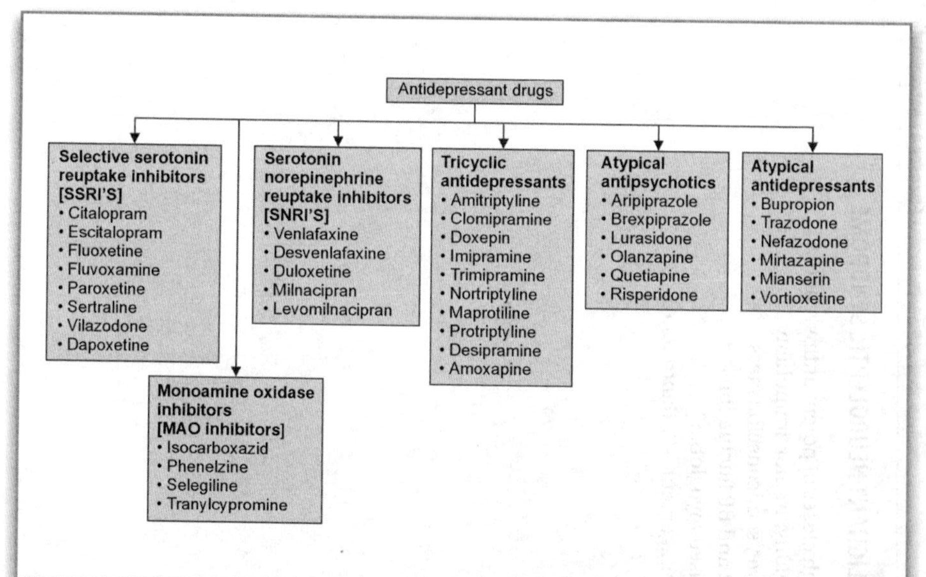
Antidepressant drugs
Selective serotonin reuptake inhibitors [SSRI'S]
• Citalopram
• Escitalopram
• Fluoxetine
• Fluvoxamine
• Paroxetine
• Sertraline
• Vilazodone
• Dapoxetine
Monoamine oxidase inhibitors [MAO inhibitors]
• Isocarboxazid
• Phenelzine
• Selegiline
• Tranylcypromine
Serotonin norepinephrine reuptake inhibitors [SNRI'S]
• Venlafaxine
• Desvenlafaxine
• Duloxetine
• Milnacipran
• Levomilnacipran
Tricyclic antidepressants
• Amitriptyline
• Clomipramine
• Doxepin
• Imipramine
• Trimipramine
• Nortriptyline
• Maprotiline
• Protriptyline
• Desipramine
• Amoxapine
Atypical antipsychotics
• Aripiprazole
• Brexpiprazole
• Lurasidone
• Olanzapine
• Quetiapine
• Risperidone
Atypical antidepressants
• Bupropion
• Trazodone
• Nefazodone
• Mirtazapine
• Mianserin
• Vortioxetine

5 CHAPTER

Antidepressant Drugs

TRICYCLIC ANTIDEPRESSANTS (TCAs)

DCP	**DESI**	**ANTI**
Doxepin	**D**ESI pramine	**A**mitriptyline
Clomipramine		**N**ortriptyline
Protriptyline		**T**rimipramine
		Imipramine

MOA: Inhibit active reuptake of amine (5HT, DA, NA)

↓

Increase concentration of amines in synaptic cleft

↓

Stimulative action (DA) and antidepressive action (NA, 5HT)

C/I of TCAs: **GEEP**

Glaucoma

Epilepsy

Enlarged **P**rostate

Uses: **DEPRESSION**

Depression

Enuresis
Photophobia
Recurrent panic attacks
Eating disorders
Smoking cessation (Bupropion)
Stress disorder (post-traumatic)
Impulsive disorder (kleptomania)
Obsessive compulsive disorder
Neuropathic pain

A/E: **TCAS**
Tremors
Cvs arrhythmias
Anticholinergic side effect
Sedation, seizure

SELECTIVE SEROTONIN REUPTAKE INHIBITORS (SSRIs)

PSE Full **C**orrect
Paroxetine
Sertraline
Escitalopram
Fluoxetine
Citalopram

MOA: Selectively inhibit membrane associated serotonin transporter

S/E: **SSRI**
Serotonin syndrome
Stimulate CNS

Reproductive dysfunction in male
Insomnia

Uses:

1. Depression
2. Obsessive compulsive disorder
3. Post-traumatic stress disorder
4. Bulimia
5. Premenstrual tension syndrome
6. Panic disorder

SNRI: Serotonin and noradrenalin reuptake inhibitors
Venlafaxine, duloxetine

ATYPICAL ANTIDEPRESSANTS

BATT

Bupropion
Amineptine
Tianeptine
Trazodone

Uses:

DONE PAPAM
Depression
Obsessive compulsive disorders
Neuropathic pain
Enuresis
Pruritus
Anxiety disorders
Phobic State
Attention deficit disorders in children
Migraine

MAO A INHIBITORS

- Moclobemide
- Clorgyline

D/I of MAO I:

1. Serotonin syndrome—if SSRI and MAO I given
2. Cheese reaction—MAOI and food rich in tyramine

Uses:

- Depression SSRI preferred over TCA
- Panic disorder
- Obsessive compulsive disorder
- Nocturnal enuresis
- Prophylaxis of migraine
- C/C pain including neuralgia
- Atopic dermatitis

DOC for bulimia—SSRI.
DOC for retarded depression—trazadone.
DOC for nocturnal enuresis—imipramine.
DOC for smoking cessation—bupropion.
DOC for peripheral neuropathy—lamotrigine.
DOC for sleep walking—carbamazepine.

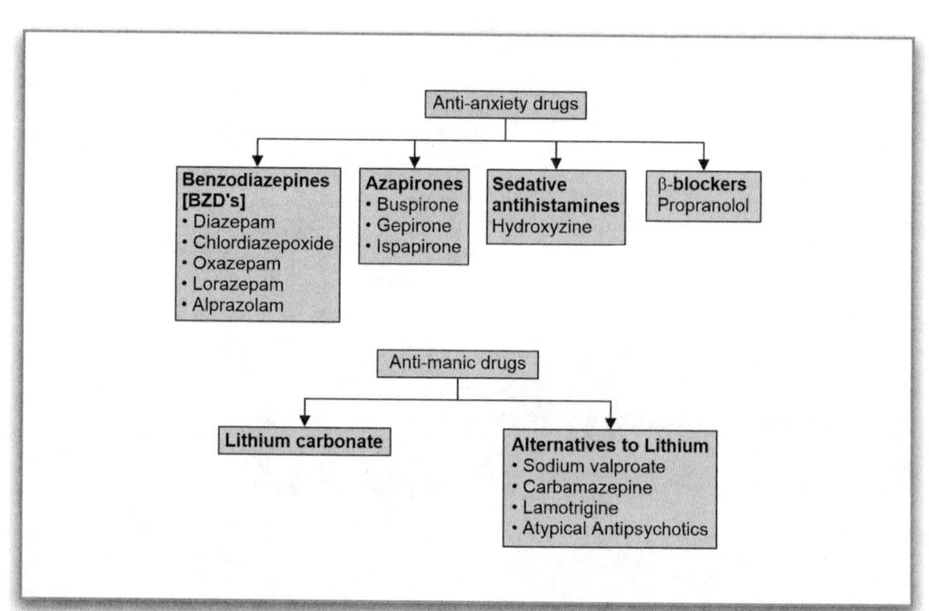

Anti-anxiety drugs
Benzodiazepines [BZD's]
• Diazepam
• Chlordiazepoxide
• Oxazepam
• Lorazepam
• Alprazolam
Azapirones
• Buspirone
• Gepirone
• Ispapirone
Sedative antihistamines
Hydroxyzine
β-blockers
Propranolol
Anti-manic drugs
Lithium carbonate
Alternatives to Lithium
• Sodium valproate
• Carbamazepine
• Lamotrigine
• Atypical Antipsychotics

6 CHAPTER

Antianxiety and Antimanic Drugs

ANTIANXIETY DRUGS

a. Benzodiazepines **A COLD**
   - **A**lprazolam
   - **C**hlordiazepoxide
   - **O**xazepam
   - **L**orazepam
   - **D**iazepam

b. Azapirones **BIG**
   - **B**uspirone
   - **I**psapirone
   - **G**epirone

c. Sedative antihistaminic—hydroxyzine

d. β-blocker—propranolol

ANTIMANIC DRUGS

- Lithium
- Sodium valproate
- Carbamazepine
- Topiramate
- Atypical antipsychotics

- Benzodiazepines

S/E: **LITHIUM**

Low therapeutic index—hence TDM essential
Increased **T**remors
Hypothyroidism
Increased **U**rine
Moms beware (teratogenic)

DOC for achieving selective antianxiety effect without sedation—buspirone.
DOC for sedation and hypnosis in patient with severe liver disease—lorazepam/oxazepam.
DOC for panic disorders—alprazolam.

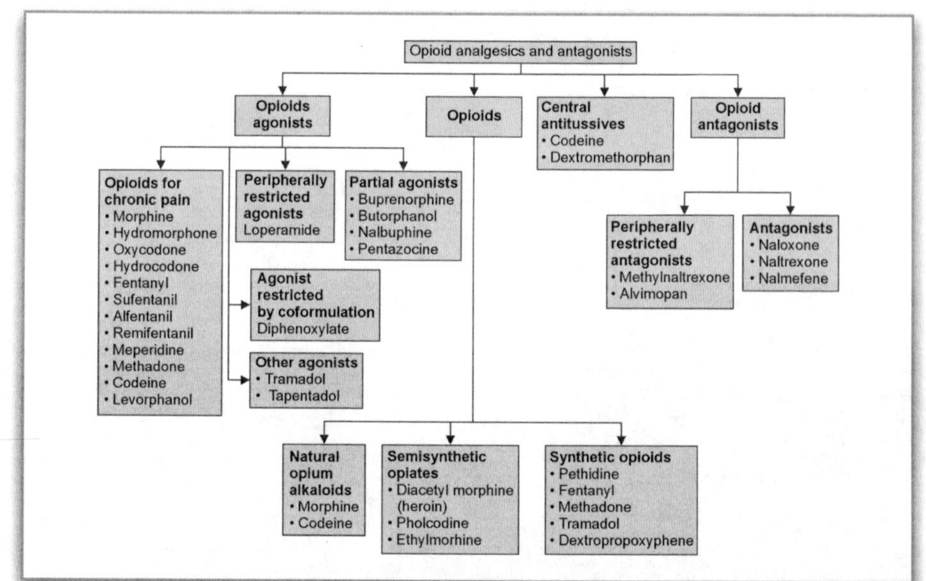

Opioid analgesics and antagonists
Opioids agonists
Opioids
Central antitussives
• Codeine
• Dextromethorphan
Opioid antagonists
Opioids for chronic pain
• Morphine
• Hydromorphone
• Oxycodone
• Hydrocodone
• Fentanyl
• Sufentanil
• Alfentanil
• Remifentanil
• Meperidine
• Methadone
• Codeine
• Levorphanol
Peripherally restricted agonists
Loperamide
Partial agonists
• Buprenorphine
• Butorphanol
• Nalbuphine
• Pentazocine
Agonist restricted by coformulation
Diphenoxylate
Other agonists
• Tramadol
• Tapentadol
Peripherally restricted antagonists
• Methylnaltrexone
• Alvimopan
Antagonists
• Naloxone
• Naltrexone
• Nalmefene
Natural opium alkaloids
• Morphine
• Codeine
Semisynthetic opiates
• Diacetyl morphine (heroin)
• Pholcodine
• Ethylmorhine
Synthetic opioids
• Pethidine
• Fentanyl
• Methadone
• Tramadol
• Dextropropoxyphene

7

CHAPTER

Opioid Analgesics

- Opioid agonist
  - Natural opium alkaloid — Morphine, codeine
  - Semisynthetic — Heroin, pholcodine
  - Synthetic — Pethidine, tramadol, Methadone, fentanyl
- Opioid agonist-antagonist — Nalorphine, pentazocine, butorphanol
- Partial M receptor agonist — Buprenorphine
- Pure opioid antagonists — Naloxone, naltrexone, nalmefene

Action of morphine: **MARPHINE CVS**

Miosis
Analgesis-**A**nalgesic
Respiratory depression
Physical and psychologic dependence
Histamine release
Itching
Nausea vomiting-stimulating
Euphoria
Cough suppression, constipation-cough and diarrhea

Vagal stimulation
Sedation and hypnosis—anxiety

C/I of Morphine:

- Head injury, undiagnosed A/C abdomen
- Bronchial asthma, COPD
- Hypotensive state, hypothyroidism
- Infants and elderly

DOC for opioid of choice in biliary spasm—pethidine.
DOC for opioid withdrawal—methadone.
DOC for C/C cancer pain—morphine.
DOC for pain of AMI—morphine.
DOC for morphine poisoning—naloxone.

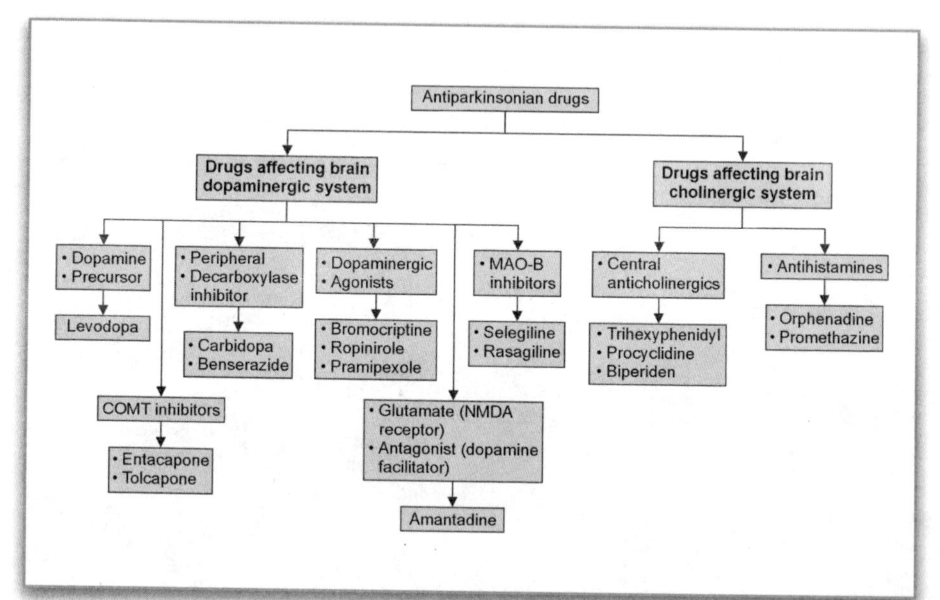
Antiparkinsonian drugs
Drugs affecting brain dopaminergic system
Drugs affecting brain cholinergic system
• Dopamine
• Precursor
Levodopa
COMT inhibitors
• Entacapone
• Tolcapone
• Peripheral
• Decarboxylase inhibitor
• Carbidopa
• Benserazide
• Dopaminergic
• Agonists
• Bromocriptine
• Ropinirole
• Pramipexole
• Glutamate (NMDA receptor)
• Antagonist (dopamine facilitator)
Amantadine
• MAO-B inhibitors
• Selegiline
• Rasagiline
• Central anticholinergics
• Trihexyphenidyl
• Procyclidine
• Biperiden
• Antihistamines
• Orphenadine
• Promethazine

8 CHAPTER

Antiparkinsonian Drugs

1. DRUGS INFLUENCING BRAIN DOPAMINERGIC SYSTEM

a. Dopamine precursor	Levodopa
b. Dopamine agonist	Bromocriptine
Ropinirole	
c. Dopamine releasing agent	Amantadine
d. MAO-B inhibitors	Selegiline
e. COMT inhibitors	Tolcapone Entacapone
f. Peripheral decarboxylase inhibitor	Carbidopa Benserazide

2. DRUGS AFFECTING BRAIN CHOLINERGIC SYSTEM

a. Central anticholinergics	Benzhexol, benztropine Procyclidine
b. Antihistaminic	Orphenadrine, promethazine

Levodopa

MOA: Transported to CNS and converted to dopamine

Uses: Parkinsonism and for restless leg syndrome
S/E: Postural hypotension, cardiac arrhythmia and exacerbation of angina

Entacapone

MOA:
- Inhibits COMT in periphery
- Reduces the metabolism of levodopa

S/E: Hepatotoxicity

Benztropine

Antagonist at M receptors in basal ganglia—reduce tremor and rigidity.

DOC for Parkinson disease—Levodopa.
DOC for drug-induced PD—Anticholinergic drugs/benzhexol.
DOC for motor fluctuation caused by levodopa—Amantadine.
DOC for neuropathic pain—Lamotrigine.
DOC for trigeminal neuralgia—Carbamazepine/gabapentin.
DOC for reducing alcohol craving—Naltrexone.

BROMOCRIPTINE

MOA:
- Potent agonist of D2
- Partial agonist and antagonist action on D1

Dosage: 1.25 mg once at night and then 5–10 mg TID
Side effects: Hallucination
First dose hypotension

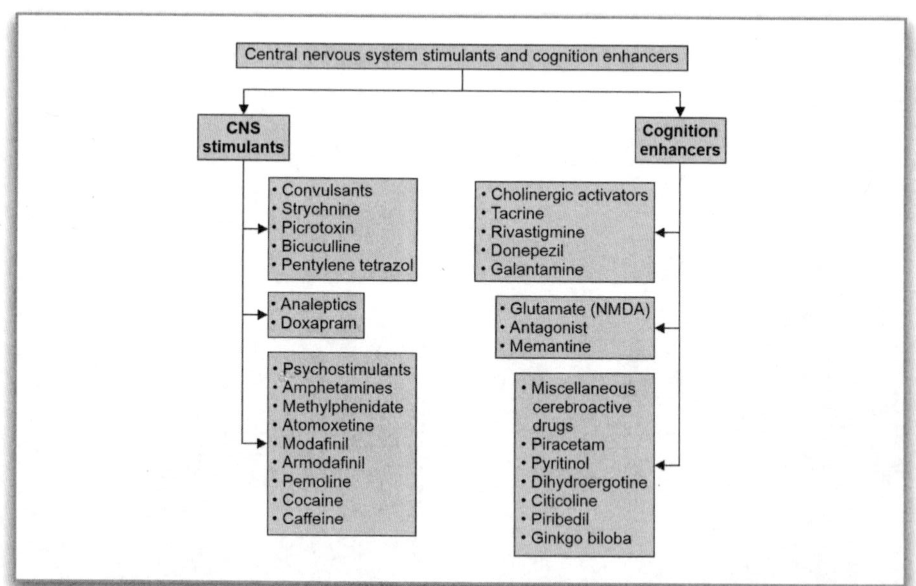

Central nervous system stimulants and cognition enhancers
CNS stimulants
Cognition enhancers
• Convulsants
• Strychnine
• Picrotoxin
• Bicuculline
• Pentylene tetrazol
• Analeptics
• Doxapram
• Psychostimulants
• Amphetamines
• Methylphenidate
• Atomoxetine
• Modafinil
• Armodafinil
• Pemoline
• Cocaine
• Caffeine
• Cholinergic activators
• Tacrine
• Rivastigmine
• Donepezil
• Galantamine
• Glutamate (NMDA)
• Antagonist
• Memantine
• Miscellaneous cerebroactive drugs
• Piracetam
• Pyritinol
• Dihydroergotine
• Citicoline
• Piribedil
• Ginkgo biloba

9

CHAPTER

Central Nervous System Stimulants and Cognition Enhancers

CLASSIFICATION

Convulsants	Strychnine, picrotoxin, bicuculline
Analeptics	Doxapram
Psychostimulants	Amphetamines, methylphenidate, modafinil, pemoline, cocaine, caffeine.

Analeptics

MOA: Stimulate respiratory centers.

Uses:
- Hypnotic drug poisoning.
- Suffocation on drowning.
- Apnea in premature infants.

AMPHETAMINES

MOA:
- Central sympathomimetics
- Causes alertness, increased concentration, attention span and working capacity

Uses:
- Night shift workers
- Antiobesity drug

COGNITION ENHANCERS (CEREBROACTIVE DRUGS)

Indications:
- Dementia (Alzheimer's)
- Mental retardation, learning defect
- Attention deficit disorder
- Transient Ischemic attacks

MOA:
- Increased cerebral blood flow
- Enhance neurotransmission
- Improvement of discrete cerebral functions, e.g. memory

C/S:
- Cholinergic activators—rivastigmine, donepezil, galantamine, tacrine
- NMDA antagonist—memantine
- Miscellaneous—piracetam, pyritinol, ginkgo biloba

DOSAGE OF DRUGS IN CNS

Disulfiram	1 g on 1st day, 0.75 g on 2nd and so on
Fomepizole	15 mg/g IV 10 mg/kg every 12 hours—methanol poisoning
Ethanol	0.7 mL/kg, nasogastric tube, 0.15 mL/kg/drip-methanol
Phenobarbitone	30–60 mg oral OD-TDS, 100–200 mg IM/IV 60 mg daily, 3–6 mg/kg—seizure
Zolpidem	5–10 mg at bedtime
Zaleplon	5–10 mg
Melatonin	3 mg at evening time

Dextropropoxyphene	60–120 mg oral
Tramadol	50–100 oral/IM/slow IV
Pentazocine	50–100 mg oral, 30–60 mg IM/SC
Butorphanol	1–4 mg IM/IV—postoperative pain
Naloxone	0.4–0.8 mg/IV antagonize morphine
Naltrexone	50 mg/day
Doxapram	40–80 mg IV/IM
Methylphenidate	5–10 mg BD
Modafinil	100–200 mg—for daytime sleep
Rivastigmine	1.5 mg BD
Donepezil	5 mg OD HS
Galantamine	4 mg BD
Memantine	5 mg OD

2

SECTION

Drugs Acting on Peripheral Nervous System

- Skeletal Muscle Relaxants
- Local Anesthetics

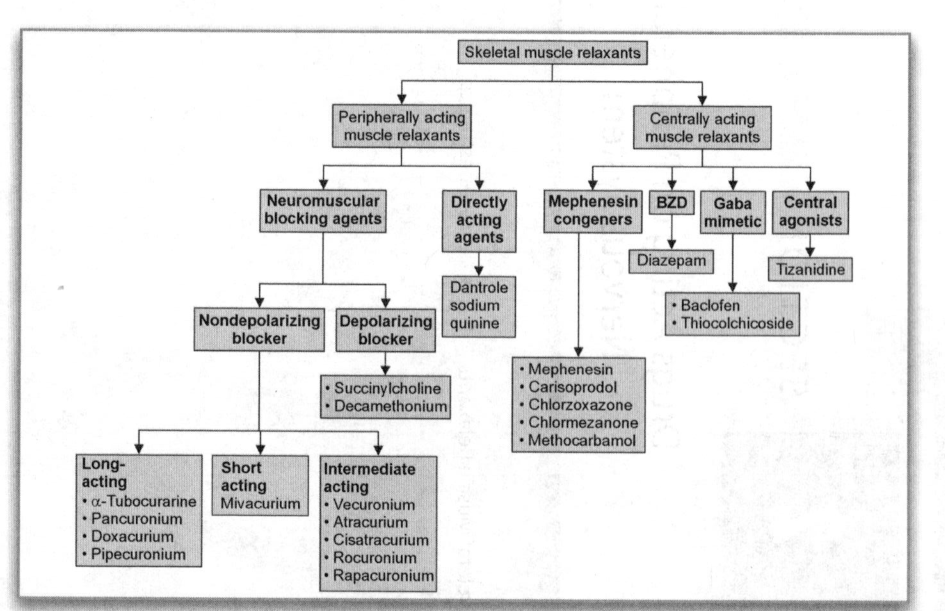

Skeletal muscle relaxants
Peripherally acting muscle relaxants
Centrally acting muscle relaxants
Neuromuscular blocking agents
Directly acting agents
Mephenesin congeners
BZD
Gaba mimetic
Central agonists
Diazepam
Tizanidine
Dantrole sodium quinine
• Baclofen
• Thiocolchicoside
Nondepolarizing blocker
Depolarizing blocker
• Succinylcholine
• Decamethonium
• Mephenesin
• Carisoprodol
• Chlorzoxazone
• Chlormezanone
• Methocarbamol
Long-acting
• α-Tubocurarine
• Pancuronium
• Doxacurium
• Pipecuronium
Short acting
Mivacurium
Intermediate acting
• Vecuronium
• Atracurium
• Cisatracurium
• Rocuronium
• Rapacuronium

CHAPTER 10

Skeletal Muscle Relaxants

PERIPHERALLY ACTING

Neuromuscular Blocking Agent

1. **Nondepolarizing**

Long acting	d-Tubocurarine
	Pancuronium—in neurosurgery
Intermediate	Vecuronium spontaneous recovery, Cardiovascular stability
	Atracurium Hofmann elimination and spontaneous degradation
Short acting	Mivacurium—shortest acting NMB

2. **Depolarizing** Succinylcholine—shortest acting SMR

Directly Acting Agent

Dantrolene sodium

Uses:
- Orally in upper motor neuron lesion (UMNL)
- Hemiplegia
- Paraplegia
- Cerebral palsy

	– Multiple sclerosis
	– IV—malignant hyperthermia
A/E:	Muscle—weakness
	Sedation
	Troublesome diarrhea
	Liver toxicity
Quinine	Used in patient with nocturnal leg cramps

CENTRALLY ACTING

♦ Mephenesin congeners	Mephenesin	
	Carisoprodol	
♦ Benzodiazepines	Diazepam	
♦ GABA derivative	Baclofen	
♦ Central α_2 agonist	Tizanidine	
MOA:	NMJ blockers	Inhibit NM receptor
	Dantrolene	Act on RyR receptor—Prevent Ca^{2+} release
	Centrally acting	Depress spinal and supraspinal Polysynaptic reflex

Uses:

1. Adjuvant to GA
2. Assisted ventilation
3. In convulsions
4. Severe case of tetanus, status Epilepticus

A/E:

1. Respiratory paralysis
2. Prolonged apnea

3. Fall in BP and cardiovascular collapse
4. Cardiac arrhythmias and arrest

DOC for short procedure laryngoscopy and bronchoscopy—Succinylcholine
DOC for muscle relaxation in hepatic and renal failure patients—Atracurium
DOC for producing relaxation in asthma patient—Pancuronium
DOC for reduction of spasticity in multiple sclerosis—Baclofen
DOC for producing relaxation for short duration surgery—Mivacurium

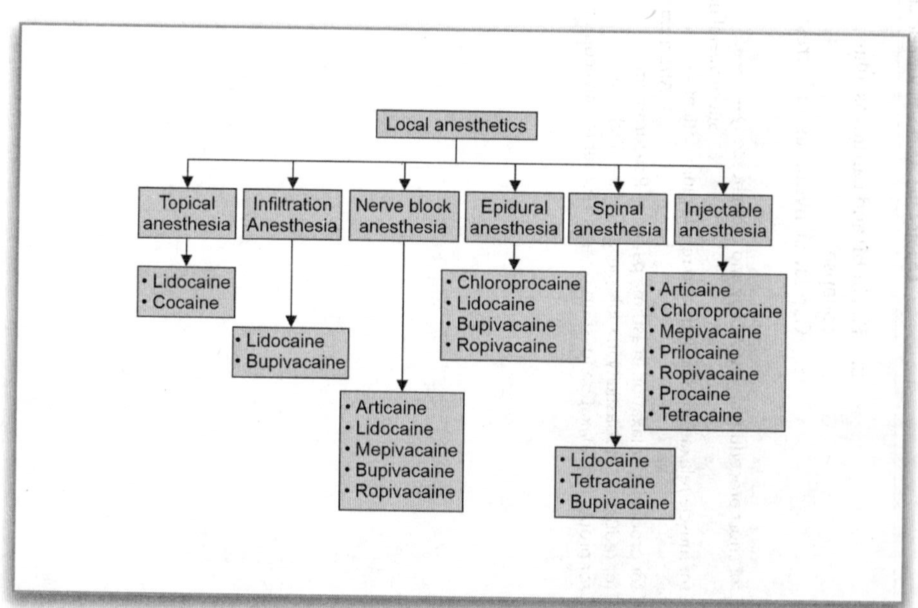
Local anesthetics
Topical anesthesia
• Lidocaine
• Cocaine
Infiltration Anesthesia
• Lidocaine
• Bupivacaine
Nerve block anesthesia
• Articaine
• Lidocaine
• Mepivacaine
• Bupivacaine
• Ropivacaine
Epidural anesthesia
• Chloroprocaine
• Lidocaine
• Bupivacaine
• Ropivacaine
Spinal anesthesia
• Lidocaine
• Tetracaine
• Bupivacaine
Injectable anesthesia
• Articaine
• Chloroprocaine
• Mepivacaine
• Prilocaine
• Ropivacaine
• Procaine
• Tetracaine

11

CHAPTER

Local Anesthetics

CLASSIFICATION

1. INJECTABLE ANESTHETICS

Low potency, short duration	Procaine Chloroprocaine—see antiarrhythmic
Intermediate potency and duration	Lignocaine Prilocaine
High potency, long duration	Tetracaine—topical only Bupivacaine in obstetrics S/E. prolong QTC interval, ventricular tachycardia and cardiac arrest

2. SURFACE ANESTHETICS

Soluble
- Cocaine
- Lidocaine
- Tetracaine
- Benoxinate

Insoluble
- Benzocaine
- Oxethazaine

MOA: LA block nerve conduction by blocking Na^+ channel during upstroke of action potential.

Uses:

1. Surface anesthesia	Spray of lignocaine
2. Infiltration anesthesia	Lignocaine, bupivacaine
3. Conduction block	Lignocaine (1–2%), bupivacaine
4. Spinal anesthesia	Lignocaine (1–2%), Bupivacaine, tetracaine
5. Epidural anesthesia	Lignocaine, bupivacaine (0.25%)

A/E:

CNS—light headedness, dizziness
CVS—bradycardia, hypotension, cardiac arrhythmia
HS—Angioedema, rash, anaphylaxis

D-tubocurarine	0.2–0.4 mg/kg
Pancuronium	0.04–0.1 mg/kg
Doxacurium	0.03–0.08 mg/kg
Pipecuronium	0.05–0.08 mg/kg
Vecuronium	0.08–0.01 mg/kg
Atracurium	0.3–0.6 mg/kg
Cisatracurium	0.15–0.2 mg/kg
Rocuronium	0.6–0.9 mg/kg
Mivacurium	0.07–0.15 mg/kg
Succinyl choline	0.5–0.8 mg/kg
Dantrolene	25–100 mg QID-reduce spasticity in UMN disorder hemiplegia, paraplegia 1 mg/kg repeated
Quinine	200–300 mg at bedtime—nocturnal leg cramps
Carisoprodol	350 mg TDS—muscle spasm

Chlorzoxazone	500 mg TDS
Chlormezanone	100–200 mg TDS
Methocarbamol	500 mg TDS
Diazepam	5 mg TDS orally, 10–40 mg N in tetany
Baclofen	10 mg BD to 25 mg TDS

DOC for producing local anesthesia—lignocaine
DOC for obstetrical procedures—bupivacaine
DOC for LA-induced cardiac arrhythmias—esmolol

DRUGS ACTING ON AUTONOMIC NERVES SYSTEM

Parasympathetic		*Sympathetic*
Cranial outflow—3, 7, 9, 10		Thoracolumbar outflow T_1-L_3
Sacral outflow s_2 s_3 s_4		
Parasympathetic actions	*Organ*	*Sympathetic actions*
• Decrease heart rate • Decrease force of contraction	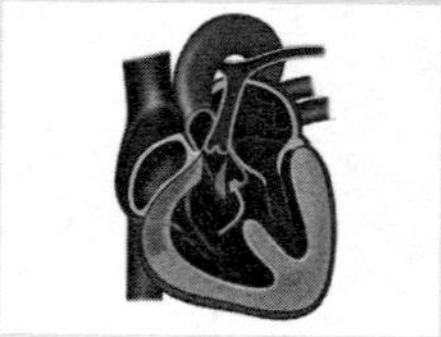 Heart	• Increase heart rate • Increase force of contraction
Decrease blood pressure	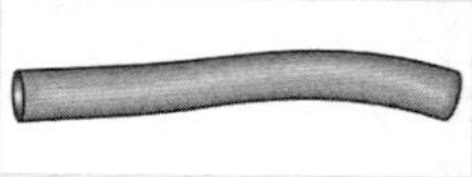 Blood vessels	Increase blood pressure
Miosis	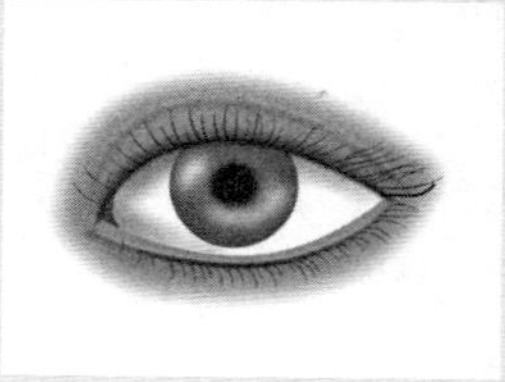 Eyes	Mydriasis

Contd...

Contd...

Bronchospasm	Bronchi	Bronchodilation
GIT motility increases and sphincters are relaxed	Gastrointestinal tract	GI motility decreases and sphincters are contracted

3

SECTION

Drugs Acting on Autonomic Nervous System

- Cholinergic System
- Adrenergic System

12 CHAPTER

Cholinergic System

CLASSIFICATION

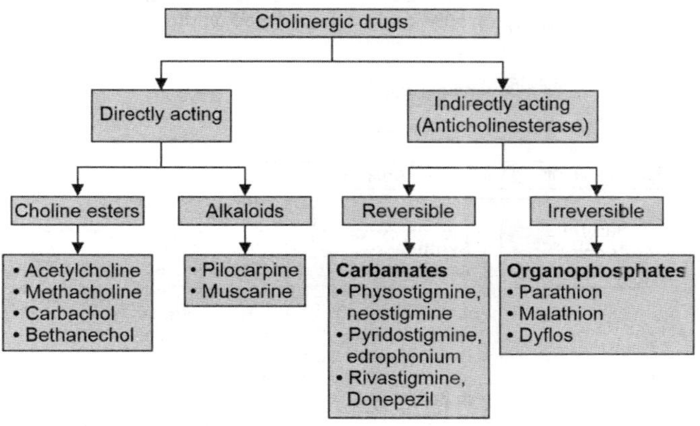

DRUGS FOR TREATING GLAUCOMA

Drugs	*Angle closure glaucoma*	*Open angle glaucoma*
Miotics	Pilocarpine (2%)	Pilocarpine (0.5%)
PGS	Latanoprost (0.005%)	Latanoprost (0.005%)
β-blockers	Timolol (0.5%) Betaxolol (0.25%)	Timolol (0.25%)
CA inhibitors	Acetazolamide	Dorzolamide (2%) Acetazolamide
Osmotic agent	Mannitol (20%) IV	Alpha: Adrenergic agonist dipivefrine (0.1%)
	Glycerol (50%) oral	Apraclonidine (1%)

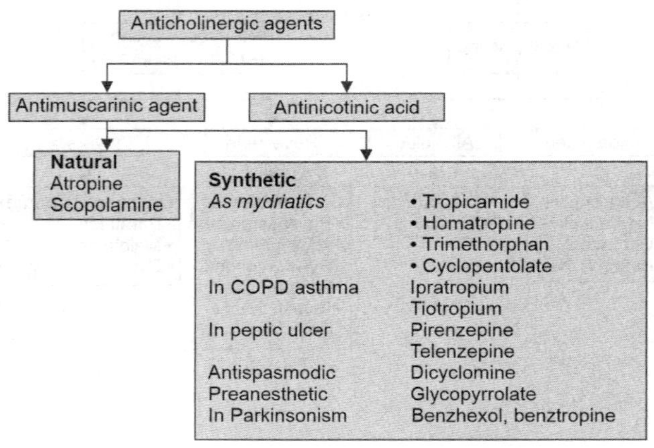

Ganglionic stimulant	
Nicotinic agonist	Nicotine
	Lobeline
Muscarinic agonist	Acetylcholine
	Carbachol

ATROPINE

Uses:	***ATROPA***
	AS Mydriatics
	Travelers diarrhea
	Rapid onset mushroom poisoning
	Organo phosphorous poisoning
	Preanesthetic medication
	Arrhythmias (Bradyarrhythmia)
S/E:	***DHATURA***
	Dry mouth, difficulty in swallowing and speaking
	Hot dry skin, hypotension
	Accommodation paralysis, blurring vision
	Tachycardia
	Urinary retention and constipation
	Respiratory depression
	Acute congestive glaucoma

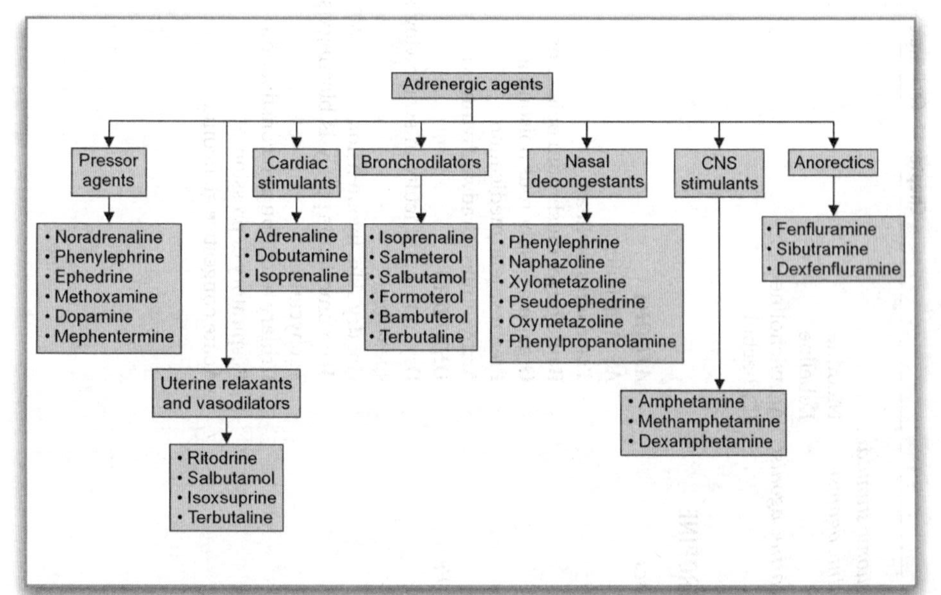

Adrenergic agents
Pressor agents
• Noradrenaline
• Phenylephrine
• Ephedrine
• Methoxamine
• Dopamine
• Mephentermine
Uterine relaxants and vasodilators
• Ritodrine
• Salbutamol
• Isoxsuprine
• Terbutaline
Cardiac stimulants
• Adrenaline
• Dobutamine
• Isoprenaline
Bronchodilators
• Isoprenaline
• Salmeterol
• Salbutamol
• Formoterol
• Bambuterol
• Terbutaline
Nasal decongestants
• Phenylephrine
• Naphazoline
• Xylometazoline
• Pseudoephedrine
• Oxymetazoline
• Phenylpropanolamine
CNS stimulants
• Amphetamine
• Methamphetamine
• Dexamphetamine
Anorectics
• Fenfluramine
• Sibutramine
• Dexfenfluramine

13 CHAPTER

Adrenergic System

SYMPATHOMIMETIC

Classification Based on their Therapeutic use

To raise BP in shock	Dopamine Ephedrine
As bronchodilator	Salbutamol, terbutaline—short acting Salmeterol, formoterol—long acting
As Cardiac stimulant	Adrenaline, isoprenaline, dopamine, dobutamine
As CNS stimulant	Modafinil, amphetamine
For local vasoconstriction	Adrenaline
For allergic reaction	Adrenaline
As nasal decongestants	Oxymetazoline, xylometazoline, Naphazoline
As anorectics	Fenfluramine, dexfenfluramine
As uterine relaxant	Salbutamol, terbutaline
As mydriatics	Ephedrine, phenylephrine
Uses of adrenaline:	**ABCDEFG** **A**naphylactic shock—0.3–0.5 mL of 1: 1000 sol IM

Bronchial asthma—0.3–0.5 mL of 1: 1 000 sol SC
Cardiac resuscitation
Duration of local anesthesia
Improved
Epistaxis control
For **G**laucoma

SYMPATHETIC BLOCKERS

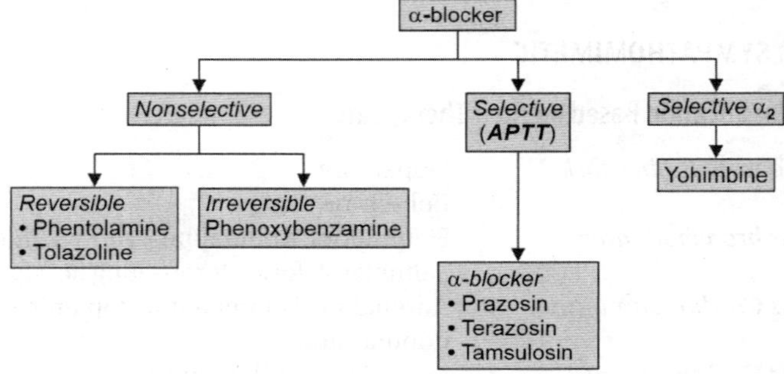

(**Tamstream D:** Tamsulosine 0.4 mg + Dutasteride 0.5 mg)

Uses of α-blocker: **MALE BPH**
Male sexual dysfunction
Benign prostatic hyperplasia
Pheochromocytoma
Hypertensive crisis

Adverse Effect

Prazosin—1st dose phenomenon—so small dose given
Tamsulosin—retrograde ejaculation

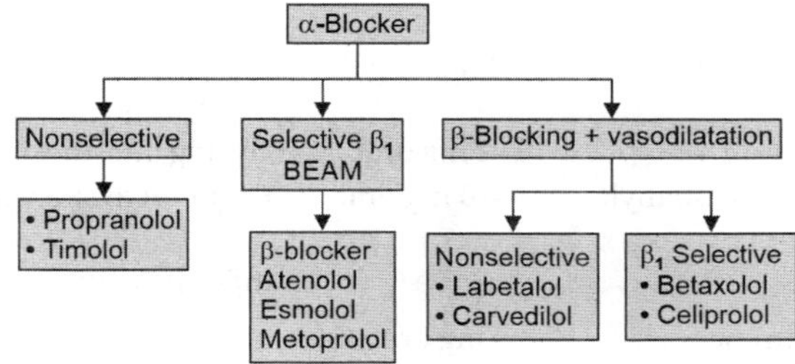

DOSAGES OF DRUGS ACTING ON ADRENERGIC SYSTEM

Bethanechol	10–40 mg oral	
Pilocarpine	0.5–4% eyedrops	
Physostigmine	0.25% eyedrops	
Hyoscine butylbromide	20–40 mg oral, IM, IV, SC	Esophageal and GI spastic conditions
Atropine methonitrate	2.5–10 mg oral, IM	Abdominal colic + hyperacidity
Ipratropium bromide	40–80 μg by inhalation	Asthma and COPD
Propantheline	15–30 mg oral	Peptic ulcer and gastritis
Oxyphenonium	5–10 mg	Peptic ulcer and GI motility

Clidinium		Nervous dyspepsia Gastritis, colic and peptic ulcer Irritable bowel syndrome
Glycopyrrolate	0.1–0.3 mg IM	Preanesthetic medication
	1–2 mg oral	During anesthesia
Pipenzolate methyl bromide	5–10 mg oral	Flatulent dyspepsia
		Infantile colic
Dicyclomine	20 mg oral/IM	
Valethamate	8 mg IM, 10 mg oral	
Oxybutynin	5 mg BD/TDS oral	
Tolterodine	2 mg BD oral	
Flavoxate	1 tab TDS	
Drotaverine	40–80 mg TDS	
Homatropine	1%, 2% eyedrops	
Cyclopentolate	0.5%, 1% eyedrops	
Tropicamide	0.5%, 1% eyedrops	
Nicotine transdermal	30 cm^2 patch	
Adrenaline	0.2–0.5 mg SC/IM repeated every 2 hours in systemic use 1 in 20,000–1 in 10,000 for local application	
Noradrenaline	2–4 μg/min IV infusion	
Isoprenaline	20 mg sublingual, 1–2 mg IM	
Dopamine	0.2–1 mg/min IV infusion	
Dobutamine	2–8 μg/kg/min IV	

Amphetamine	5–10 mg oral
Ephedrine	15–60 mg TDS
Phenylephrine	2–5 mg IM 0.1–0.5 mg slow IV
Methoxamine	10–20 mg IM, 3–5 mg slow IV
Mephentermine	10–20 mg oral, IM/slow IV
Isoxsuprine	5–10 mg oral, IM
Oxymetazoline	0.025–0.05% topical in nose
Xylometazoline	0.05–0.1% topical in nose
Pseudoephedrine	30–60 mg TDS
Phenylpropanolamine	25–50 mg TDS
Sibutramine	10 mg OD, then 15 mg OD
Phenoxybenzamine	20–60 mg/day oral
Phentolamine	5 mg IV repeated as required
Prazosin	1–4 mg BD/TDS
Terazosin	2–10 mg OD
Doxazosin	1 mg OD up to 8 mg
Tamsulosin **(Tamstream)**	0.2–0.4 mg OD
Propranolol	40–80 mg/day
Sotalol	160–480 mg/day
Timolol	10–40 mg/day
Pindolol	10–30 mg/day
Metoprolol **(Metopot)**	100–400 mg/day
Atenolol	25–100 mg/day
Acebutolol	400–1200 mg/day
Bisoprolol	2.5–10 mg/day
Labetalol	300–600 mg/day
Esmolol	0.5 mg/kg loading dose 0.05–0.2 mg/kg/min

Celiprolol	200–600 mg OD
Nebivolol	5 mg OD
Carvedilol	3.125 mg BD for 2 weeks max up to 25 mg BD—in CHF 6.25 mg BD initially max up to 25 mg BD—hypertension
Betaxolol	0.5% 1 drop in each eye BD
Levobunolol	0.5% 1 drop OD
Dipivefrine	0.1% 1 drop in each eye BD
Brimonidine	0.2% eyedrops 1 drop TDS
Latanoprost	0.005% 1 drop in each eye—OD in evening
Acetazolamide and dorzolamide	2% eyedrop IDS

4 SECTION

Cardiovascular Drugs

- Drugs Affecting Renin-Angiotensin System
- Cardiac Glycosides and Drugs for Heart Failure
- Antiarrhythmic Drugs
- Antianginal Drugs
- Antihypertensive Drugs

14 CHAPTER

Drugs Affecting Renin-Angiotensin System

ANGIOTENSIN CONVERTING ENZYME-INHIBITORS

- Captopril
- Enalapril
- Lisinopril
- Fosinopril
- Ramipril—Also inhibits local RAS

MOA:
- It inhibits formation of AT II
- Promote formation of bradykinin

Uses:
- Hypertension
- Congestive heart failure (CHF)
- Left ventricular hypertrophy (LVH)
- Acute myocardial infarction (AMI)
- Diabetic nephropathy
- Scleroderma crisis

S/E:
- Hypotension
- Hyperkalemia
- Cough, dysgeusia, rash
- Urticaria
- Angioedema
- Granulocytopenia

ANGIOTENSIN RECEPTOR BLOCKER

- Losartan
- Telmisartan **(Telmurix:** Telmisartan 40 mg + Chlorthalidone 6.25 mg/12.5 mg)
- Candesartan **(Olright)**
- Valsartan
- Irbesartan

MOA:	ARB's competitively block AT II at A_1 receptor
Uses:	– Hypertension – CHF – Myocardial infarction (MI) – Diabetic nephropathy (DN)
S/E:	Hypotension Hyperkalemia Fetopathic effect

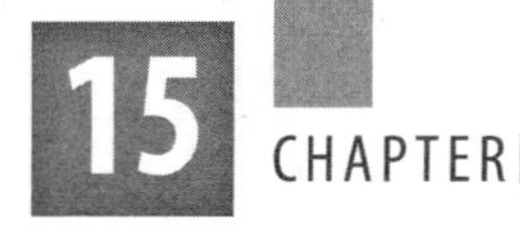

Cardiac Glycosides and Drugs for Heart Failure

CARDIAC GLYCOSIDES (CG)

Digitalis purpurea	Digitoxin
Digitalis lanata leaf	Digoxin

MOA: CG bind to extracellular face of Na^+ K^+ ATPase of myocardium-accumulation of Na^+ intracellularly. This indirectly result in intracellular Ca^{2+} accumulation and effective FOC.

Uses:

1. CHF
2. Cardiac arrhythmias
   - Atrial fibrillation
   - Atrial flutter
   - Paroxysmal supraventricular tachycardia (PSVT)

Side effects:

Low Margin of Safety

Extracardiac: Anorexia, nausea, vomiting, abdominal pain, restlessness and disorientation

Cardiac: Arrhythmia, partial to complete AV block and severe bradycardia

DRUGS FOR CONGESTIVE HEART FAILURE

♦ Inotropic agents	Digoxin Dobutamine Dopamine Milrinone
♦ Diuretics	Furosemide Thiazide Chlorthalidone
♦ Aldosterone antagonists	Spironolactone
♦ β-adrenergic blockers	Metoprolol Bisoprolol Carvedilol
♦ Vasodilators	
– Venodilators	Glyceryl trinitrate (GTN) Isosorbide dinitrate
– Arteriolar dilator	Hydralazine
– Arteriolar + Venodilator	Sodium nitroprusside
♦ Renin-angiotensin inhibitors	
ACE inhibitors	Enalapril Ramipril
Angiotensin-receptor blockers	Losartan Candesartan

Precautions and Contraindications of Cardiac Glycosides

- Hypokalemia
- Elderly, renal and hepatic failure
- Myocardial infarction
- Thyrotoxicosis
- Myxedema

- Ventricular tachycardia
- Partial AV block
- Acute myocarditis
- Wolff-parkinson-white syndrome

DOC for reducing mortality in CHF—spironolactone.
DOC for inotropic effect—dobutamine.
DOC for CHF Ist line—ACE inhibitors.
DOC for rapid diuresis—loop diuretics.

16 CHAPTER

Antiarrhythmic Drugs

CLASSIFICATION

1.	Class I	1. Procainamide Disopyramide
		2. Lignocaine MOA suppression of automaticity in ectopic foci
		3. Propafenone flecainide
2.	Class II	Propranolol Esmolol
3.	Class III	Agent widening AP—action potential Amiodarone
4.	Class IV	Calcium channel blockers Verapamil Diltiazem

Class 1

MOA:	Membrane Stabilizing agent	- Open state Na^+ channel blocker - Also delay recovery - Suppress AV conduction
Use:	VT, VF	
S/E:	50% patients develop antinuclear antibody 20% patients develop systemic lupus Erythematosus (SLE)	

Class II

MOA:	Antiadrenergic agents—suppress adrenergic-mediated ectopic activity
Use:	Treating sinus tachycardia Atrial and nodal escape

AMIODARONE

AMIODARONE
Antiarrhythmic
Multiple action—block K^+, Na^+, Ca^{2+} channel and β-receptor
Iodine containing
Orally active
Duration of action is very long (3–8 weeks)
APD and ERP increases, conduction decreases, depress ectopic
Resistant atrial fibrillation (AF), VT and recurrent VF are uses
On IV injection myocardial depression and BP fall on prolonged use causes fibrosis of lung.

Neuropathy
Eye corneal micro deposits may occur
Inhibits T_4-T_3 conversion

LIGNOCAINE

LIGNOCAINE
Local anesthetic
Inactive orally so...
Given IV for antiarrhythmic action
Na⁺ channel blocking which occur...
Only in inactive state of Na^+ channels
CNS S/E like convulsion
Action last only 15 min due to rapid redistribution
Inhibit Purkinje fibers and ventricle but...
No effect on AVN and SAN so...
Effective only in ventricular arrhythmia

DOC for ventricular tachycardia—lidocaine
DOC for ventricular fibrillation—lidocaine
DOC for sick sinus syndrome—theophylline
DOC for intraoperative arrhythmias—esmolol
DOC for PSVT—adenosine
DOC for maintenance of sinus rhythm—amiodarone
DOC for resistant recurrent AF—flecainide

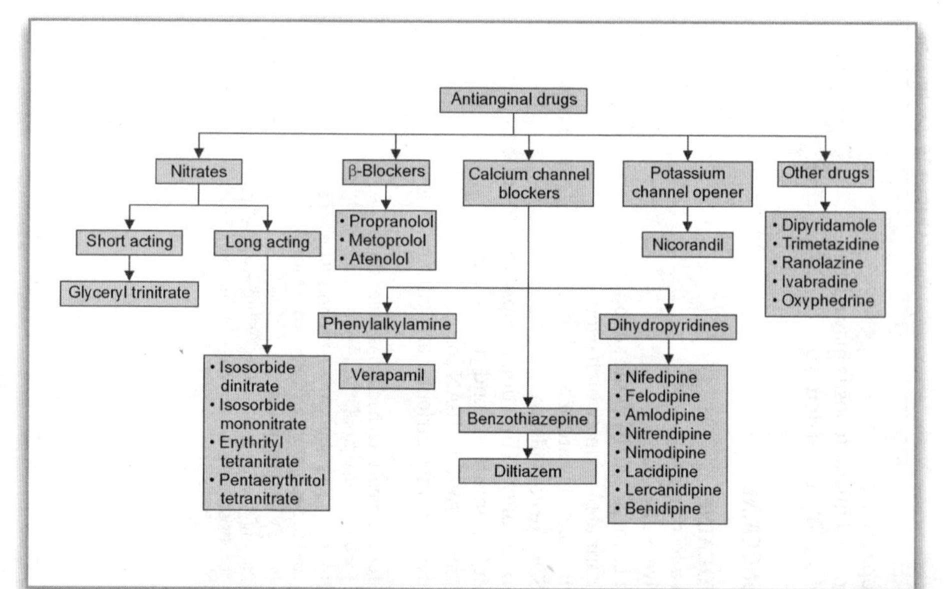
Antianginal drugs
Nitrates
β-Blockers
Calcium channel blockers
Potassium channel opener
Other drugs
Short acting
Long acting
Glyceryl trinitrate
• Isosorbide dinitrate
• Isosorbide mononitrate
• Erythrityl tetranitrate
• Pentaerythritol tetranitrate
• Propranolol
• Metoprolol
• Atenolol
Phenylalkylamine
Verapamil
Benzothiazepine
Diltiazem
Dihydropyridines
• Nifedipine
• Felodipine
• Amlodipine
• Nitrendipine
• Nimodipine
• Lacidipine
• Lercanidipine
• Benidipine
Nicorandil
• Dipyridamole
• Trimetazidine
• Ranolazine
• Ivabradine
• Oxyphedrine

17 CHAPTER

Antianginal Drugs

1.	Nitrates	Short acting	Glyceryl trinitrate
		Long acting	Isosorbide dinitrate
			Isosorbide mononitrate
			Erythrityl tetranitrate
2.	Beta-blocker **PAM**		**P**ropranolol
			Atenolol
			Metoprolol
3.	Ca^{2+} channel blocker	Phenylalkylamine	**V**erapamil—act on **V**entricle
		Benzothiazepine	Diltiazem
		Dihydropyridines	Amlodipine
			Nifedipine
			Felodipine
			Nitrendipine
4.	K^{+} channel opener		Nicorandil
5.	Others		Dipyridamole

CA^{2+} CHANNEL BLOCKER

MOA: Intracellular Ca^{2+} concentration maintains the tone of smooth muscle and myocardial contraction

- Calcium channel blockers (CCBS) block L-type calcium channel (heart and vasculature)
- Decreases intracellular Ca^{2+}
- Decreases total peripheral resistance (all CCBs)
- Decreases the cardiac output (verapamil and diltiazem—decrease contractility/HR/AV conduction)

Uses:	Hypertension (all CCBs) Angina (all CCBs)—Prinzemental angina Antiarrhythmic (verapamil and diltiazem) Peripheral vascular disease (PVD)—Raynaud's phenomenon
A/E:	Reflex tachycardia (dipines) Gingival hyperplasia (dipines) Constipation (verapamil)

NITRATE

MOA:

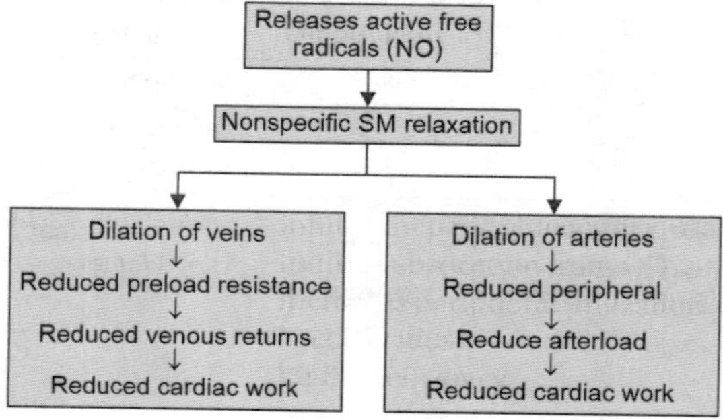

Uses:	– Angina pectoris – Acute coronary syndromes – Myocardial infarction – CHF and acute LVF – Biliary colic – Esophageal spasm – Cyanide poisoning
S/E:	Fullness in head, throbbing headache, flushing, weakness, methemoglobinemia

DOC for acute attack of angina—Nitrates
DOC for variant angina—Diltiazem

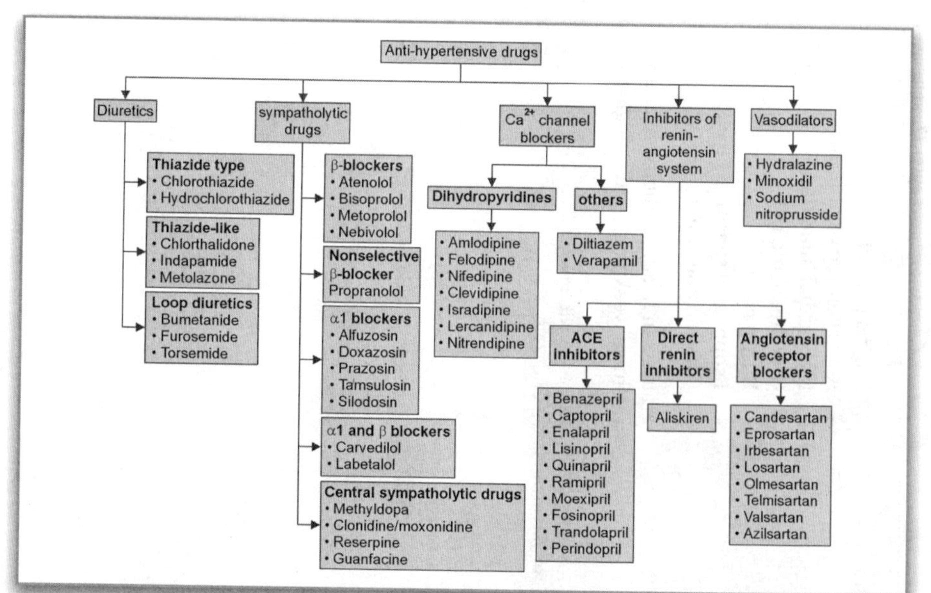

Anti-hypertensive drugs
Diuretics
Thiazide type
• Chlorothiazide
• Hydrochlorothiazide
Thiazide-like
• Chlorthalidone
• Indapamide
• Metolazone
Loop diuretics
• Bumetanide
• Furosemide
• Torsemide
sympatholytic drugs
β-blockers
• Atenolol
• Bisoprolol
• Metoprolol
• Nebivolol
Nonselective β-blocker
Propranolol
α1 blockers
• Alfuzosin
• Doxazosin
• Prazosin
• Tamsulosin
• Silodosin
α1 and β blockers
• Carvedilol
• Labetalol
Central sympatholytic drugs
• Methyldopa
• Clonidine/moxonidine
• Reserpine
• Guanfacine
Ca^{2+} channel blockers
Dihydropyridines
• Amlodipine
• Felodipine
• Nifedipine
• Clevidipine
• Isradipine
• Lercanidipine
• Nitrendipine
others
• Diltiazem
• Verapamil
Inhibitors of renin-angiotensin system
ACE inhibitors
• Benazepril
• Captopril
• Enalapril
• Lisinopril
• Quinapril
• Ramipril
• Moexipril
• Fosinopril
• Trandolapril
• Perindopril
Direct renin inhibitors
Aliskiren
Angiotensin receptor blockers
• Candesartan
• Eprosartan
• Irbesartan
• Losartan
• Olmesartan
• Telmisartan
• Valsartan
• Azilsartan
Vasodilators
• Hydralazine
• Minoxidil
• Sodium nitroprusside

18 CHAPTER

Antihypertensive Drugs

CLASSIFICATION

1.	Diuretics	Thiazide—hydrochlorothiazide Chlorthalidone **(Chlohat)**, indapamide High ceiling—furosemide K^+ sparing—spironolactone, amiloride
2.	ACE inhibitors	Captopril, lisinopril Enalapril, ramipril
3.	ARBs	Losartan, candesartan Valsartan, telmisartan **(Telmuix:** Telmisartan 40 mg, Chlorthalidone 6.25/12.5 mg**)**
4.	CCBs	Verapamil, diltiazem Amlodipine, felodipine, nifedipine
5.	α-adrenergic blocker	Prazosin, terazosin
6.	β-adrenergic blocker	Propranolol, atenolol

Contd ..

Contd...

7.	Central sympatholytic	Clonidine, methyldopa
8.	$\alpha + \beta$ adrenergic blocker	Labetalol, carvedilol
9.	Vasodilators	Arterial—hydralazine, minoxidil Artery + Vein—sodium nitroprusside

DOC for hypertension emergencies —sodium nitroprusside
DOC for hypertension in pregnancy—methyldopa
Male pattern baldness—minoxidil.

DOSAGE OF DRUGS USED IN CARDIOVASCULAR SYSTEM

Captopril	25–150 mg/day
Enalapril	2.5–40 mg/day
Lisinopril	5–40 mg/day
Fosinopril	10–40 mg/day
Perindopril	2–8 mg/day
Ramipril	1.25–10 mg/day
Losartan	50 mg OD
Candesartan	8 mg OD
Irbesartan	150–300 mg OD
Valsartan	80–160 mg OD 1 hour before meals
Telmisartan	20–80 mg OD
Digoxin	0.125–0.5 mg
Digitoxin	0.05–0.2 mg
Amrinone	0.5 mg/kg bolus inj
Milrinone	50 μg/kg/IV bolus
Quinidine	100–200 mg TDS
Procainamide	0.5–1 g oral/IM, 0.25–0.5 g every 2 hours
Disopyramide	100–150 mg 6–8 hourly oral
Lidocaine	50–100 mg bolus IV, followed by 20–40 mg every 10 min
mexiletine	100–200 mg IV over 10 min 150–200 mg TDS oral
Propafenone	150 mg BD—300 mg TDS
Amiodarone	100–300 mg slow IV 30–60 min 400–600 mg/day orally

Verapamil	5 mg IV over 2–3 min 60–120 mg TDS oral
Adenosine	6–12 mg rapid IV
Atropine	0.6–1.2 mg IM
Diltiazem	30–60 mg TDS–QID oral
Nifedipine	5–20 mg BD-TDS oral
Felodipine	5–10 mg OD Max of 10 mg BD
Amlodipine	5–10 mg OD
Nitrendipine	5–20 mg OD
Lacidipine	4 mg OD, increase to 6 mg OD
Nicorandil	5–20 mg BD
Dipyridamole	25–100 mg TDS
Lercanidipine	10–20 mg OD
Benidipine	4–8 mg OD
Trimetazidine	20 mg TDS
Xyphendrine	8–24 mg TDS, 4–8 mg IV OD-BD
Cyclandelate	200–400 mg TDS
Xanthinol nicotinate	300–600 mg TDS oral, 300 mg IM or slow IV
Pentoxifylline	400 mg BD-IDS
Indapamide	2.5 mg daily
Prazosin	0.5 mg at bedtime max of 10 mg BD
Clonidine	Start with 100 μg OD/BD max of 300 μg TDS orally/IM
Methyldopa	0.25–0.5 g BD-QID oral
Hydralazine	25–50 mg OD-IDS
Sodium nitroprusside	50 mg added to 500 mL of saline bottle

5

SECTION

Respiratory System Drugs

- Drugs for Cough
- Drugs for Bronchial Asthma

19 CHAPTER

Drugs for Cough

CLASSIFICATION

1.	**Pharyngeal demulcents**	Lozenges Glycerine
	MOA:	Soothing effect on throat
2.	**Expectorants**	
	Bronchial secretion enhancers	Na^+ or K^+ ctrate Potassium iodide
	Mucolytics	Bromhexine Ambroxol N-acetyl cysteine (also used in paracetamol poisoning)
	MOA:	Lysis of mucus
	S/E:	Rhinorrhea Lacrimation

Contd...

Contd...

3.	**Antitussives**	
	Opioids	Codeine, pholcodine
	Nonopioid	Noscapine, dextromethorphan
	MOA:	Depress cough center
	S/E:	Sedation Impairment of mental function
	Antihistamine	Chlorpheniramine
4.	**Adjuvant bronchodilators**	Salbutamol Terbutaline

DOC for suppression of cough—dextromethorphan.
DOC for apnea in premature infants—theophylline.
DOC for ACE inhibitor induced cough—aspirin.

20 CHAPTER

Drugs for Bronchial Asthma

BRONCHODILATOR

1. Sympathomimetic

Nonselective	• Adrenaline • Ephedrine
Short-acting β_2-agonist	• Salbutamol • Terbutaline
Long-acting β_2-agonist	• Salmeterol • Formoterol

MOA: β_2-agonist activate adenylyl cyclase which convert ATP into cAMP, which is required for smooth muscle relaxation.

2. Methylxanthines/PDEI

- Theophylline
- Aminophylline

MOA: Methylxanthines inhibit phosphodiesterase enzyme which convert cAMP into AMP.

3. Anticholinergics

- Ipratropium bromide
- Tiotropium bromide

MOA: By blocking cholinergic constrictor tone mainly acts on large bronchi.

Use:
- Asthma
- Chronic obstructive pulmonary disease (COPD)

NB: β_2-agonists act on small bronchi

ANTI-INFLAMMATORY

1. Systemic Steroids

- Hydrocortisone
- Prednisolone

2. Inhalational Steroids

- Beclomethasone
- Budesonide
- Fluticasone, flunisolide

MOA: Suppress bronchial inflammation

S/E:
- Hoarseness of voice
- Dysphonia
- Sore throat
- Oropharyngeal candidiasis

Indications of Systemic Steroids

1. Status asthmaticus
2. Chronic persistent asthma

3. Mast Cell Stabilizers

- Na$^+$ cromoglycate
- Ketotifen

MOA:	Inhibits degranulation of mast cell
Use:	Bronchial asthma Allergic rhinitis Allergic conjunctivitis

4. Leukotriene Antagonist

- Montelukast
- Zafirlukast

5. Anti-IgE Antibody

Omalizumab

> DOC for aspirin-induced asthma—leukotriene receptor antagonist.
> DOC for exercise-induced asthma—mast cell stabilizer.
> DOC for poorly controlled asthma—theophylline.
> DOC for acute attack of asthma—nebulized salbutamol.
> DOC for COPD—ipratropium bromide.

DOSAGE OF DRUGS USED IN COUGH AND ASTHMA

Bromhexine	8 mg TDS children 4 mg BD
Ambroxol	15–30 mg TDS
Carbocisteine	250–750 mg TDS
Codeine	10–30 mg, children 2–5 mg
Pholcodine	10–15 mg daily
Noscapine	15–30 mg children 7.5 mg
Dextromethorphan	10–20 mg children 2.5–5 mg
Chlorpheniramine	2–5 mg TID
Diphenhydramine	15–25 mg OD
Promethazine	15–25 mg OD
Salbutamol	2–4 mg oral, 0.25–0.5 mg IM/SC 100–200 μg by inhalation
Terbutaline	5 mg oral, 0.25 mg SC, 250 μg by inhalation
Bambuterol	10–20 mg single evening dose
Salmeterol	25 μg/metered dose inhaler 2 puffs BD
Formoterol	12–24 μg by inhalation twice daily
Theophylline	100–300 mg TDS
Aminophylline	250–500 mg oral/slow IV
Montelukast	10 mg OD
Zafirlukast	20 mg BD
Ketotifen	1–2 mg BD
Corticosteroid inhaled	100–200 μg BD start up to 400 μg QID
Systemic steroid—prednisolone	20–60 mg/day-start

6 SECTION

Gastrointestinal Drugs

- Antiemetic Drugs
- Drugs for Peptic Ulcer
- Antidiarrheal Agents

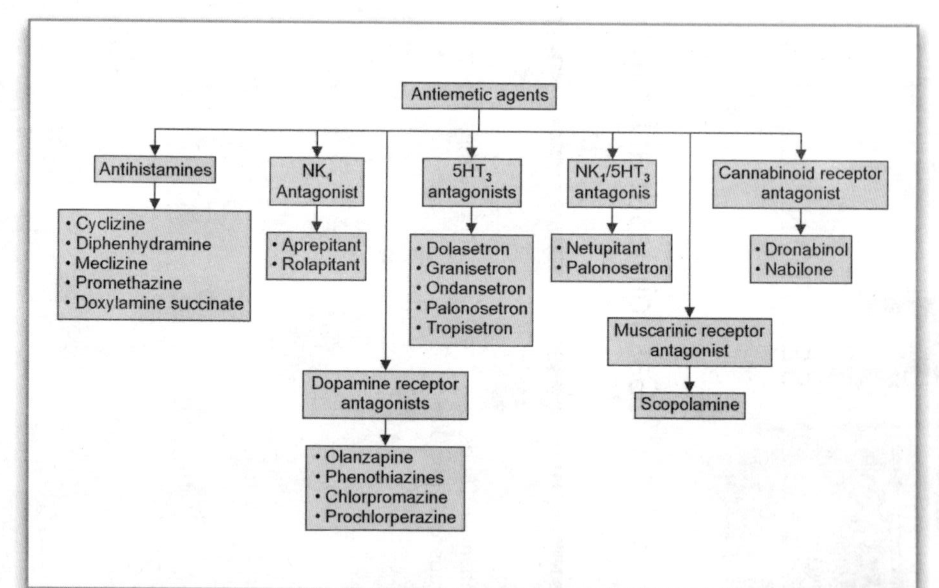

Antiemetic agents
Antihistamines
• Cyclizine
• Diphenhydramine
• Meclizine
• Promethazine
• Doxylamine succinate
NK1 Antagonist
• Aprepitant
• Rolapitant
5HT3 antagonists
• Dolasetron
• Granisetron
• Ondansetron
• Palonosetron
• Tropisetron
NK1/5HT3 antagonis
• Netupitant
• Palonosetron
Cannabinoid receptor antagonist
• Dronabinol
• Nabilone
Dopamine receptor antagonists
• Olanzapine
• Phenothiazines
• Chlorpromazine
• Prochlorperazine
Muscarinic receptor antagonist
Scopolamine

21 CHAPTER

Antiemetic Drugs

CLASSIFICATION

Antiemetics	*Examples*	*Use*	*S/E*
Anticholinergics	Hyoscine Dicyclomine	Motion sickness	Dry mouth, sedation
Antihistamine	Dimenhydrinate Diphenhydramine Promethazine	Motion sickness Meniére's disease Drug-induced vomiting	Dry mouth
5 HT_3 receptor antagonist	Ondansetron Granisetron	GERD Intractable hiccups Chemotherapy-induced vomiting	 Headache, dizziness, diarrhea

Contd...

Contd...

Prokinetic agents	Metoclopramide Domperidone (Preferred)	Drug-induced vomiting	• EPS Gynecomastia • Rare EPS (Extra-pyramidal S/E)
Chlorpromazine neuroleptics	Chlorpromazine Haloperidol	Drug-induced vomiting	Extrapyramidal S/E
Cannabinoids	Dronabinol	Radiation induced	• Sedation • Euphoria • Hallucination

MOA:

Anticholinergic	Block afferent impulse from vestibular apparatus to vomiting center
Antihistaminics	Sedative and central anticholinergic action
$5HT_3$ receptor	Block vagal afferent from gut to CTZ and STN
Prokinetic	Block 5 HT_3 and D2 in CTZ and D2 in basal ganglia—EPS
Neuroleptics	Block D2 receptors in CTZ

DOC for nausea and vomiting—metoclopramide.
DOC for D2 blockers (Haloperidol)-induced EPS—promethazine.

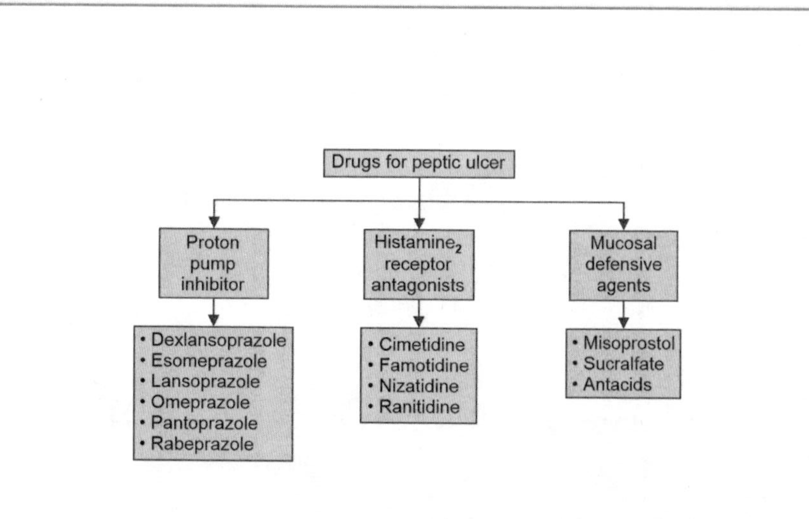

Drugs for peptic ulcer
Proton pump inhibitor
Histamine$_2$ receptor antagonists
Mucosal defensive agents
• Dexlansoprazole
• Esomeprazole
• Lansoprazole
• Omeprazole
• Pantoprazole
• Rabeprazole
• Cimetidine
• Famotidine
• Nizatidine
• Ranitidine
• Misoprostol
• Sucralfate
• Antacids

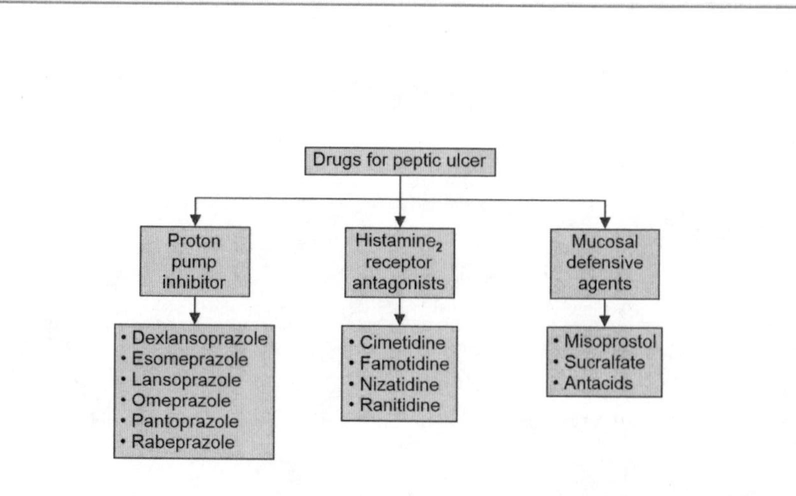

Drugs for peptic ulcer
Proton pump inhibitor
Histamine2 receptor antagonists
Mucosal defensive agents
• Dexlansoprazole
• Esomeprazole
• Lansoprazole
• Omeprazole
• Pantoprazole
• Rabeprazole
• Cimetidine
• Famotidine
• Nizatidine
• Ranitidine
• Misoprostol
• Sucralfate
• Antacids

22 CHAPTER

Drugs for Peptic Ulcer

CLASSIFICATION

1. DRUGS THAT INHIBIT GASTRIC ACID SECRETION

a. Proton pump inhibitors—Ex**PLOR**	**O**meprazole **R**abeprazole **P**antoprazole **L**ansoprazole **E**someprazole
b. H_2 receptor antagonist	Cimetidine Ranitidine Famotidine
c. Antimuscarinic agents	Pirenzepine Telenzepine
d. PG analogues	Misoprostol

2. ULCER PROTECTIVE

- Sucralfate
  MOA: It precipitates surface and dietary protein at ulcer base and acts as physical barrier.
- Colloidal bismuth subcitrate (CBS)

3. NEUTRALIZE GASTRIC ACID

Systemic	Sodium bicarbonate
	Sodium citrate
Nonsystemic	Magnesium hydroxide S/E diarrhea
	Aluminum hydroxide S/E constipation

4. ANTI-*HELICOBACTER PYLORI* DRUGS

Pumba **ATM** **C**losed

- **P**PIs
- **A**moxicillin
- **T**etracycline
- **M**etronidazole
- **C**BS

Proton Pump Inhibitors (PPIs)

MOA:	PPIs bind covalently with SH gp of the H^+, K^+ ATPase enzyme-irreversibly inhibit it
Uses:	All Peptic ulcer disease
	GERD
	Zollinger-Ellison syndrome
A/E:	Decreased vitamin B_{12} absorption
	Risk of infection on chronic use—gastric tumor

H_2 Receptor Antagonist

MOA:	H_2 receptor blocker—competitively block H_2 receptor
Uses:	H_2 blockers are used preoperatively

S/E:	Cimetidine—enzyme inhibitor, cross BBB, antiandrogenic—it cause gynecomastia and female pattern of hair growth so now replaced by other H_2 receptor blockers (Ranitidine).

PG Analogues

S/E:	Diarrhea and abdominal cramps
MOA:	Inhibiting acid secretion and promote mucus and HCO_3—secretion, inhibit gastrin production
Indications:	NSAID-associated GI injury and blood loss

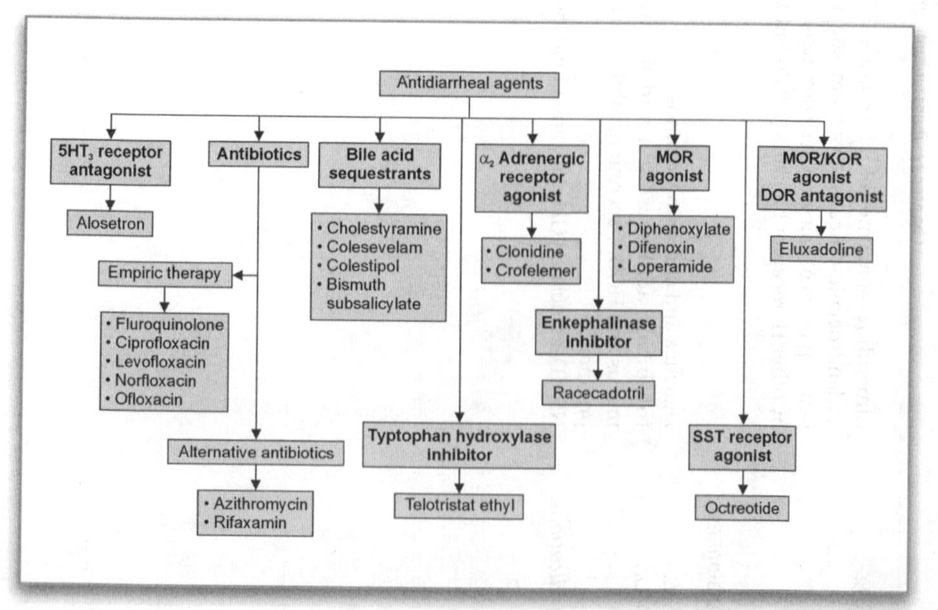
Antidiarrheal agents
5HT$_3$ receptor antagonist
Alosetron
Antibiotics
Empiric therapy
• Fluroquinolone
• Ciprofloxacin
• Levofloxacin
• Norfloxacin
• Ofloxacin
Alternative antibiotics
• Azithromycin
• Rifaxamin
Bile acid sequestrants
• Cholestyramine
• Colesevelam
• Colestipol
• Bismuth subsalicylate
Typtophan hydroxylase inhibitor
Telotristat ethyl
α_2 Adrenergic receptor agonist
• Clonidine
• Crofelemer
Enkephalinase inhibitor
Racecadotril
MOR agonist
• Diphenoxylate
• Difenoxin
• Loperamide
SST receptor agonist
Octreotide
MOR/KOR agonist DOR antagonist
Eluxadoline

23 CHAPTER

Antidiarrheal Agents

CLASSIFICATION

1. NONSPECIFIC THERAPY

A. Oral and parenteral rehydration
B. **Antimotility and antisecretory agents:**
   - Opioids—codeine, loperamide,
   - Adrenergic—receptor agonist: Clonidine
   - Octreotide

2. SPECIFIC THERAPY (ANTIBIOTICS)

SECS—Ciprofloxacin 500 mg BD × 5 days
- ***S**higella*
- ***E**. coli*
- ***C**ampylobacter jejuni*
- ***S**almonella*

VCD
***V**ibrio **C**holera—**D**oxycycline* 100 mg BD × 5 days

ECG—Metronidazole
- *Entamoeba histolytica*—400 mg TDS × 7 days

- *Clostridium difficile*—800 mg TDS × 10 days
- *Giardia lamblia*—200 mg TDS × 5 days

LAXATIVES

♦ *Bulk laxatives*	Dietary fiber
♦ *Stool softeners*	**L**iquid paraffin
Use:	**L**ubricant effect
S/E:	**L**ipid pneumonia
	Leakage of fecal matter
	Long-term—use causes deficiency of fat soluble vitamins (A, D, E, K)
♦ *Stimulant laxatives*	Phenolphthalein
	Bisacodyl
♦ *Osmotic laxative*	Magnesium sulfate
	Sodium sulfate
	Lactulose
♦ *HT4 agonist*	Prucalopride

DOC for functional diarrhea—loperamide.
DOC for diabetic diarrhea—clonidine.
DOC for secretory diarrhea—cholestyramine.
DOC for hepatic encephalopathy—lactulose.

DOSAGE OF DRUGS

Ranitidine	300 mg at bedtime/150 mg BD for ulcer healing
	150 mg at bed time—maintenance
Famotidine	40 mg at bedtime/20 mg BD for ulcer healing
Roxatidine	150 mg at bed time/75 mg BD
Omeprazole	20–40 mg OD for peptic ulcer
	60–120 mg/day 2 divided doses—ZE syndrome
	20–60 daily—GERD
Esomeprazole	20–40 mg OD
Lansoprazole	15–30 mg OD
Pantoprazole **(Panpot)**	40 mg OD
Rabeprazole **(Rabipot)**	20 mg OD, 60 mg/day—ZE syndrome
Misoprostol	200 μg QID
Hyoscine	0.2–0.4 mg oral/IM
Dicyclomine	10–20 mg oral
Metoclopramide	1 mg/kg IV—antiemetic
Domperidone	10–40 mg TDS
Mosapride	5 mg TDS
Ondansetron	8 mg oral, 4 mg IV
Granisetron	10 μg/kg IV 30 min before chemotherapy
	2 mg oral–1 hour before chemotherapy

Methyl polysiloxane	40–120 mg 3–4 times a day
Docusates	100–400 mg/day
	50–150 mg in 50–100 mL—as enema
Phenolphthalein	60–130 mg/day
Bisacodyl	5–15 mg/day
Sodium picosulfate	5–10 mg at bedtime
Tegaserod	2–6 mg BD before meals
Lactulose	109 BD with plenty of water
	20 g TDS—hepatic encephalopathy
Mesalazine	2.4 g/day—ulcerative colitis
Racecadotril	100 mg TDS
Diphenoxylate	5–10 mg, followed by 2.5–5 mg 6th hourly
Loperamide	4 mg followed by 2 mg after each motion

7 SECTION

Drugs Acting on Kidney

- Diuretics and Antidiuretics

24 CHAPTER

Diuretics and Antidiuretics

CLASSIFICATION

High efficacy diuretics: Furosemide
Torsemide **(Toracor)**

MOA: Inhibit Na^{+}– K^{+}– 2Cl co-transport

Site: Thick ascending loop of Henle

A/E: **DHHA**
Dil. Hyponatremia
Hypokalemia
Hearing loss
Acute saline depletion

Moderate efficacy: Thiazide
Chlorothiazide
Hydrochlorothiazide
Polythiazide
Clopamide
Indapamide
Xipamide

Use: **DHHE**

Diabetes insipidus
Hypercalciuria
Hypertension
Edema

MOA: Inhibit Na^+ Cl symport
Site: Early DT
A/E: Same as above

Low efficacy K^+ sparing

Spironolactone
Amiloride
Triamterene

S/E: **GIM**

Gynecomastia
Impotence
Menstrual irregularities

Carbonic anhydrase inhibitors

Acetazolamide
Dorzolamide

MOA: Inhibit carbonic anhydrase in proximal tubules
Uses: Epilepsy
Periodic paralysis
Acute mountain sickness
Glaucoma
To alkalinize urine

S/E: Acidosis, hypokalemia, drowsiness and hepatic coma

Osmotic Diuretics **GIMU**

Glycerol
Isosorbide
Mannitol
Urea

Uses: Increased intracranial tension
To maintain GFR and urine flow
To counteract low osmolarity of plasma

DOC for edema in CHF/renal failure/cirrhosis—Furosemide.
DOC for cerebral edema—Mannitol.
DOC for thiazide-induced hypokalemia—Spironolactone.
DOC for idiopathic hypercalciuria—Thiazides.
DOC for lithium-induced nephropathy—Amiloride.

ANTIDIURETICS

Drugs Reducing Urine Volume

A. *Vasopressin:* Secreted from post pituitary
Release via V1 and V2 receptors

Action: Vasoconstriction—raise blood pressure
Urine retention

Analogues: Desmopressin
Terlipressin
Lypressin

Uses: Diabetes insipidus
Hemophilia
Esophageal varices

B. Thiazides
C. Chlorpropamide (OHA-sensitize kidney to ADH action)
D. Carbamazepine—stimulate ADH secretion

DOSAGE OF DRUGS USED IN RENAL SYSTEM

Drug	Dosage
Furosemide	20–80 mg/daily in morning—in renal failure
Bumetanide	1–5 mg oral OD in morning, 2–4 mg IV/IM
Torsemide **(Toracor)**	2.5–5 mg OD—Hypertension
	5–20 mg/day—in edema up to 100 mg in RF
Hydrochlorothiazide	12.5–100 mg/day
Benzthiazide	25–100 mg/day
Hydroflumethiazide	25–100 mg/day
Chlorthalidone	50–100 mg/day
Metolazone	5–20 mg/day
Xipamide	20–40 mg/day
Indapamide	2.5–5 mg/day
Clopamide	10–60 mg/day
Acetazolamide	250 mg OD-BD
Spironolactone	25–50 mg BD-QID
Triamterene	50–100 mg daily
Amiloride	5–10 mg OD-BD
Mannitol	1–1.5 g/kg infused
Lypressin	10 IU IM/SC or 20 IU dil in 200 mL of dextrose solution
Terlipressin	2 mg IV repeat 1–2 mg every 40–60 hours
Desmopressin	Intranasal 10–40 μg/day in 2–3 divided doses oral 0.1–0.2 mg TDS, 2–4 μg/day SC/IV

8 SECTION

Autacoids and Related Drugs

- Antihistaminics
- Serotonin and Drugs for Migraine
- Prostaglandins
- Nonsteroidal Anti-inflammatory Drugs
- Antirheumatoid and Antigout Drugs

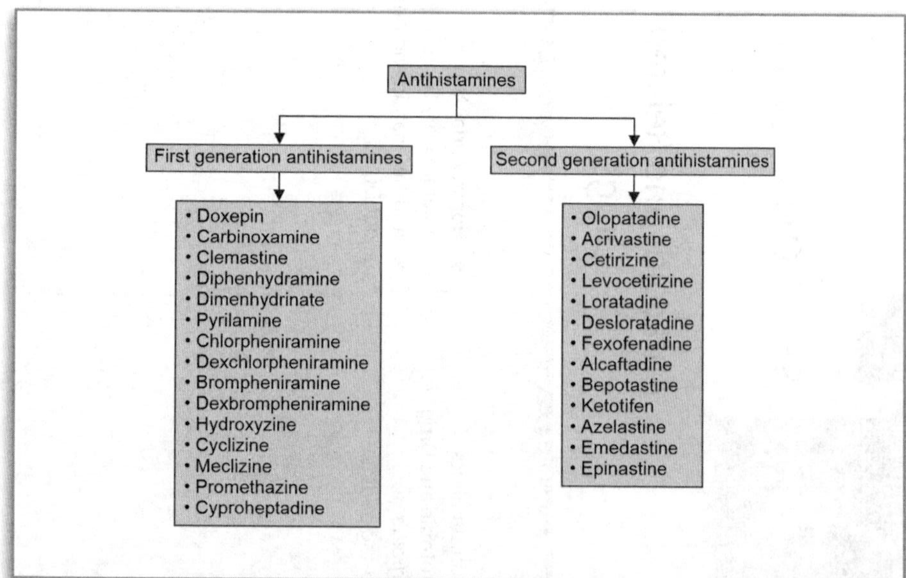
Antihistamines
First generation antihistamines
• Doxepin
• Carbinoxamine
• Clemastine
• Diphenhydramine
• Dimenhydrinate
• Pyrilamine
• Chlorpheniramine
• Dexchlorpheniramine
• Brompheniramine
• Dexbrompheniramine
• Hydroxyzine
• Cyclizine
• Meclizine
• Promethazine
• Cyproheptadine
Second generation antihistamines
• Olopatadine
• Acrivastine
• Cetirizine
• Levocetirizine
• Loratadine
• Desloratadine
• Fexofenadine
• Alcaftadine
• Bepotastine
• Ketotifen
• Azelastine
• Emedastine
• Epinastine

25 CHAPTER

Antihistaminics

CLASSIFICATION

First Generation

- Diphenhydramine
- Dimenhydrinate
- Promethazine
- Cinnarizine
- Pheniramine

  MOA: Competitively blocking H1 receptor.

  Uses: Allergic D, common cold, Preanesthetic medi, antiemetics, parkinsonism, sedative and hypnotics.

  S/E: CNS depression-sedation, dryness of mouth, blurring of vision, constipation, urinary retention.

Second Generation

Cetirizine
Levocetirizine **(Zeez)**; **(Zeez M**: Levocetirizine 5 mg + Montelukast 10 mg**)**
Loratadine
Fexofenadine
Azelastine

MOA: Block H1 receptor selectively

Uses: Allergic condition—rhinitis
Dermatitis
Conjunctivitis
Urticaria
Eczema

ANTIVERTIGO DRUGS

- Cinnarizine
- Promethazine
- Hyoscine
- Diazepam
- Amitriptyline.

DOC for rhinorrhea—fexofenadine, cetirizine.

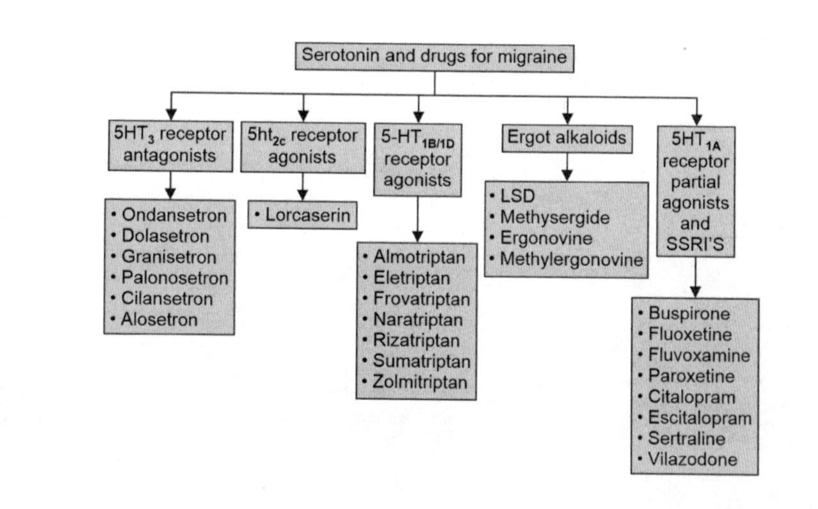
Serotonin and drugs for migraine
$5HT_3$ receptor antagonists
• Ondansetron
• Dolasetron
• Granisetron
• Palonosetron
• Cilansetron
• Alosetron
$5ht_{2c}$ receptor agonists
• Lorcaserin
$5\text{-}HT_{1B/1D}$ receptor agonists
• Almotriptan
• Eletriptan
• Frovatriptan
• Naratriptan
• Rizatriptan
• Sumatriptan
• Zolmitriptan
Ergot alkaloids
• LSD
• Methysergide
• Ergonovine
• Methylergonovine
$5HT_{1A}$ receptor partial agonists and SSRI'S
• Buspirone
• Fluoxetine
• Fluvoxamine
• Paroxetine
• Citalopram
• Escitalopram
• Sertraline
• Vilazodone

26 CHAPTER

Serotonin and Drugs for Migraine

CLASSIFICATION

Agonist	MOA
Buspirone	5 HT_{1A} partial agonist
Triptans	Selective 5 $HT_{IB/ID}$ agonist
Ergotamine	Partial agonist at $5HT_1$
Metoclopramide	$5HT_4$ agonist
Antagonist	MOA
Ketanserin	$5HT_4$ antagonist
Cyproheptadine	$5HT_{2A}$ antagonist
Methysergide	$5HT_{2A}$ antagonist
Ondansetron	$5HT_{2A/2C}$ antagonist
Granisetron	$5HT_3$ antagonist

DRUGS FOR MIGRAINE

Mild	Analgesic + NSAIDs + Antiemetics
Moderate	NSAIDs + Ergot alkaloid + Antiemetics
Severe	Sumatriptan + Ergot alkaloid + Antiemetic

Sumatriptan

MOA:	5HT 1B/1D receptor agonist
Uses:	Migraine

	Suppress neurogenic inflammation of cranial nerves
S/E:	Tightening of head and chest Bradycardia Coronary vasospasm Risk of myocardial infarction

DOC for serotonin syndrome—cyproheptadine.
DOC for acute attack of migraine—sumatriptan.

27 CHAPTER

Prostaglandins

PROSTAGLANDINS

MEDICAL

Dinoprostone	Induction of labor, mid-term abortion, termination of pregnancy
Carboprost	Mid-term abortion, control of PPT
Alprostadil	Maintain PDA, erectile dysfunction
Misoprostol	Peptic ulcer, abortion, PPI+
Epoprostenol	
Iloprost	Pulmonary hypertension
Latanoprost	Glaucoma

Actions—**PG**

Pyrexia
Peripheral nerve sensitization
Peripheral and pulmonary artery resistance reduced
PDA maintained
Pulmonary hypertension reduced
Priming of cervix before labor
Postpartum hemorrhage control
Platelet aggregation prevented
Promote healing of peptic ulcer

Peristalsis increased
Purging effect (diarrhea)
To control erectile dysfunction
Glaucoma

DOC for cushing's syndrome and meningioma—mifepristone.

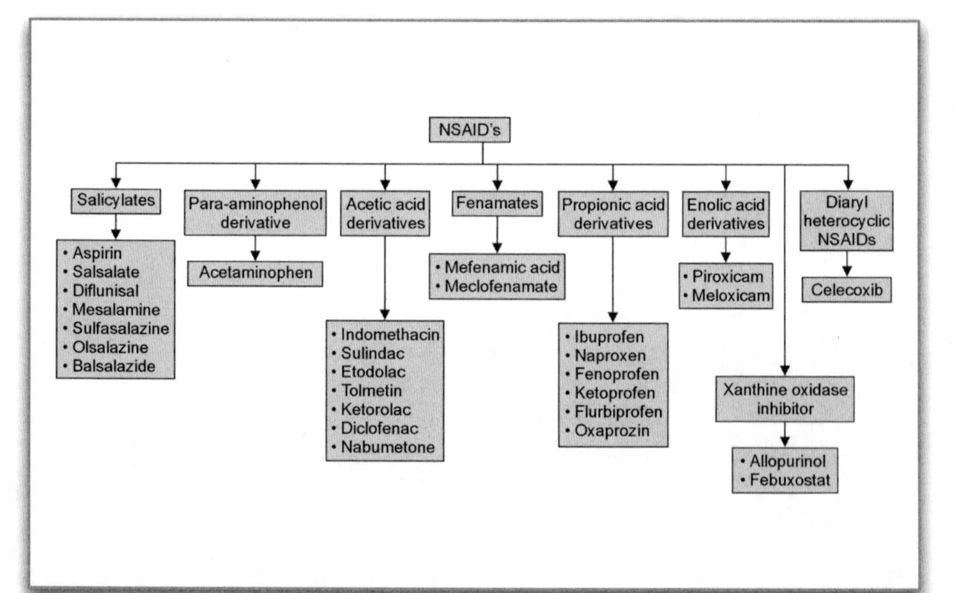

NSAID's
Salicylates
• Aspirin
• Salsalate
• Diflunisal
• Mesalamine
• Sulfasalazine
• Olsalazine
• Balsalazide
Para-aminophenol derivative
Acetaminophen
Acetic acid derivatives
• Indomethacin
• Sulindac
• Etodolac
• Tolmetin
• Ketorolac
• Diclofenac
• Nabumetone
Fenamates
• Mefenamic acid
• Meclofenamate
Propionic acid derivatives
• Ibuprofen
• Naproxen
• Fenoprofen
• Ketoprofen
• Flurbiprofen
• Oxaprozin
Enolic acid derivatives
• Piroxicam
• Meloxicam
Xanthine oxidase inhibitor
• Allopurinol
• Febuxostat
Diaryl heterocyclic NSAIDs
Celecoxib

28 CHAPTER

Nonsteroidal Anti-inflammatory Drugs

CLASSIFICATION

NONSELECTIVE COX INHIBITORS

a. Salicylates	Aspirin
b. Propionic acid derivatives	Ibuprofen Ketoprofen
c. Aryl acetic acid derivatives	Diclofenac Aceclofenac (**Zyclonac P:** Aceclofenac 100 mg + Paracetamol 325 mg)
d. Anthranilic acid derivatives	Mefenamic acid
e. Pyrrolo pyrrole derivatives	Ketorolac
f. Oxicam derivatives	Piroxicam Tenoxicam
g. Indole derivatives	Indomethacin

PREFERENTIAL COX 2 INHIBITORS

- Nimesulide
- Nabumetone

HIGHLY SELECTIVE COX 2 INHIBITOR

- Celecoxib
- Etoricoxib
- Parecoxib

ANALGESIC, ANTIPYRETIC WITH POOR ANTI-INFLAMMATION

- Paracetamol
- Nefopam

MOA: Inhibition of cyclooxygenase enzyme inhibit PG and thromboxane synthesis

Uses:
- As analgesic
- As antipyretic
- Rheumatoid arthritis
- Acute rheumatic fever
- Osteoarthritis
- Thromboembolic disorders MI

A/E:
- HS—angioneurotic edema, bronchospasm (Aspirin-induced)
- GIT—dyspepsia, epigastric pain
- Bleeding
- Reye's syndrome—if associated viral infection.

DOC for paracetamol poisoning—Acetylcysteine.
DOC for aspirin poisoning—Vitamin K.
DOC for closure of patent ductus arteriosus—Indomethacin.
DOC for pain and fever—Paracetamol.

29 CHAPTER

Antirheumatoid and Antigout Drugs

DRUGS USED IN GOUT

Acute Gout

- NSAID
- *Colchicine:* Indomethacin, diclofenac, piroxicam
- *Glucocorticoids:* Prednisolone, methylprednisolone

Colchicine

MOA: Inhibit migration of granulocyte to the affected joint and thereby inhibiting the inflammatory cycle

Uses: For treating acute gout and for prophylaxis.

S/E: **MAAA** (on chronic use)
Myopathy
Alopecia's
Aplastic anemia
Agranulocytosis
Overdose—kidney damage
CNS depression
Intestinal bleeding

Long-term Control of Gout

Uricosuric Agent

- Probenecid
- Sulfinpyrazone
- Benzbromarone

Probenecid

MOA: Increase uric acid excretion and reduces its blood level

Uses: C/C gout, hyperuricemia and to prolong penicillin and ampicillin action

S/E: Dispepsia

Uric Acid Synthesis Inhibitors

Febuxostat **(Febufix)**

MOA: Selective Xanthine oxidase inhibitor

Allopurinol

MOA: Xanthine oxidase inhibitor

Uses: DOC in C/C gout—for both over producers and under excretors

Secondary hyperuricemia:

To potentiate 6 mercaptopurine in cancer chemotherapy

S/E (allopurinol):
- HS Rash
- Erythema, itching, Stevens-Johnson syndrome
- Hepatotoxicity

DRUGS USED IN RHEUMATOID ARTHRITIS

Disease **M**odifying **A**nti**R**heumatic **D**rugs (DMARDs) **MEDICALS R G**old

Methotrexate
Etanercept
d penicillamine
Infliximab
Chloroquine
Anakinra
Leflunomide
Sulfasalazine
Rituximab
Gold compound

Methotrexate

MOA: Dihydrofolate reductase inhibitor—prominent immunosuppression and anti-inflammation by inhibit production of anti-inflammatory substance

Uses: Choriocarcinoma, rheumatoid arthritis, severe psoriasis, myasthenia gravis, C/C hepatitis.

C/I: In pregnancy, breastfeeding, liver disease, active infection, peptic ulcer

A/E: Dose dependent hepatotoxicity + bone marrow suppression

Chloroquine

MOA:	Release of lysosomal enzyme and scavenge free radical.
Uses:	Malaria and rheumatoid arthritis
A/E:	Corneal opacity and retinal damage

Sulfasalazine

MOA:	Inhibits production of superoxide and inflammatory cytokines
Uses:	Ulcerative colitis and RA
S/E:	Neutropenia and thrombocytopenia and hepatitis

Gold Compound

MOA:	Alter the function of macrophages and suppress CMI

Leflunomide

MOA:	Inhibit proliferation of activated lymphocytes Active metabolite inhibit dihydrofolate dehydrogenase and pyrimidine synthesis in actively dividing cells. Long plasma $t_{1/2}$—2 weeks Loading dose given
A/E:	Loose stool Lose of hair Leucopenia Liver transaminase elevated

DOC for urate nephropathy—allopurinol.

DOSAGE OF ANTIRHEUMATOID AND ANTIGOUT DRUGS

Betahistine	4–8 mg QID
Diphenhydramine, Dimenhydrinate	
Promethazine, Hydroxyzine	25–50 mg oral
Pheniramine, Meclizine Cyproheptadine, Cinnarizine Chlorpheniramine, Buclizine	2–4 mg oral
Dexchlorpheniramine	2 mg oral
Dimethindene	1 mg oral
Triprolidine	2.5–5 mg oral
Mebhydrolin	100–300 mg oral
Cyclizine	50 mg
Clemastine	1–2 mg
Fexofenadine	120–180 mg oral
Loratadine	10 mg oral
Desloratadine	5 mg
Cetirizine	10 mg oral
Levocetirizine **(Zeez)**	5–10 mg oral
Azelastine	4 mg oral, 0.28 intranasal
Mizolastine, ebastine, rupatadine	10 mg oral
Ergotamine	1–3 mg oral/sublingual repeat
Dihydroergotamine	2–6 mg oral, 0.5–1 mg IM repeat
Dihydroergotoxine	1–1.5 mg oral/sublingual

Sumatriptan	50–100 mg oral
Rizatriptan	10 mg/2 hours
Mifepristone	600 mg orally 2 days before
Carboprost	0.25 mg IM every 30–120 minutes
Dinoprostone	1–3 mg oral/vaginal tab
Gemeprost	1 mg/3 hourly
Alprostadil	0.5 mg dilute and infuse IV
Epoprostenol	0.5 mg
Aspirin	0.3–0.6 g 6th hourly—as analgesic
Aspirin	4–5 g/day—Acute rheumatic fever
Aspirin	3–5 g/day—Rheumatoid arthritis
Aspirin	60–100 mg/day post MI
Ibuprofen	400–600 mg TDS
Naproxen	250 mg BD-TDS
Ketoprofen	50–100 mg BD-TDS
Flurbiprofen	50 mg BD-QID
Mefenamic acid	250–500 mg TDS
Diclofenac sodium	50 mg TDS, BD, 75 mg deep IM
Aceclofenac	100 mg BD
Piroxicam	20 mg BD for 2 day, 20 mg OD
Tenoxicam	20 mg OD
Ketorolac	15–30 mg IM/IV, 4–6 hourly 10–20 mg orally
Indomethacin	0.1–0.2 mg/kg—closure of PDA
Metamizol	0.5–1.5 g orally/IM/IV
Propyphenazone	300–600 mg TDS
Nimesulide	100 mg BD
Meloxicam	7.5–15 mg OD
Nabumetone	500 mg OD

Celecoxib	100–200 mg BD
Etoricoxib	60–120 mg OD
Parecoxib	40 mg oral/IV/IM-BD
Paracetamol	0.5–1 g TDS
Nefopam	30–60 mg TDS oral
Methotrexate	7.5–15 mg weekly
Azathioprine	50–150 mg/day
Sulfasalazine	1–3 g/day
Chloroquine	150 mg/day
Hydroxychloroquine	400 mg/day for 4–6 weeks 200 mg OD maintenance
Leflunomide	100 mg/day for 3 days 20 mg OD maintenance
Auranofin	6 mg/day in 1/2 doses
d-Penicillamine	125–250 mg OD then 250 mg BD
Etanercept	50 mg weekly SC inj
Infliximab	3–5 mg/kg IV every 4–8 weeks
Adalimumab	40 mg SC every 2 weeks
Anakinra	100 mg SC daily
Corticosteroids–Prednisolone	5–10 mg/day
Colchicine	1 mg orally, then 0.25 mg 1–3 hourly till control attack
Probenecid	Start 0.25 g BD max up to 0.5 g
Sulfinpyrazone	100–200 mg BD
Allopurinol	Start 100 mg OD, increase to 300 mg/day

9 SECTION

Hormones and Related Drugs

- Thyroid Hormones and Thyroid Inhibitors
- Insulin and Oral Hypoglycemic Agents
- Corticosteroids
- Androgens
- Estrogens
- Drugs Acting on Uterus
- Drugs Affecting Calcium Balance

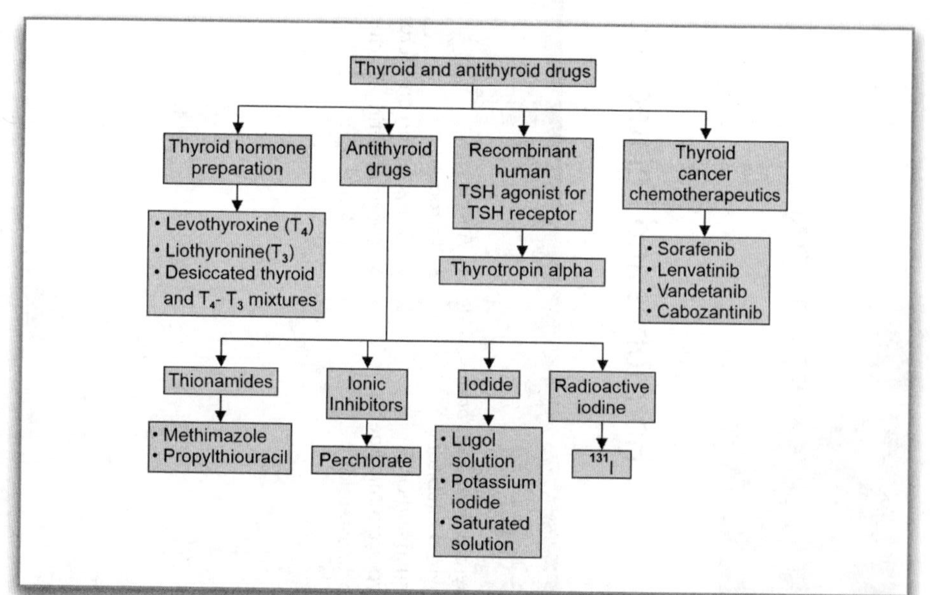
Thyroid and antithyroid drugs
Thyroid hormone preparation
Antithyroid drugs
Recombinant human TSH agonist for TSH receptor
Thyroid cancer chemotherapeutics
• Levothyroxine (T_4)
• Liothyronine(T_3)
• Desiccated thyroid and T_4- T_3 mixtures
Thyrotropin alpha
• Sorafenib
• Lenvatinib
• Vandetanib
• Cabozantinib
Thionamides
Ionic Inhibitors
Iodide
Radioactive iodine
• Methimazole
• Propylthiouracil
Perchlorate
• Lugol solution
• Potassium iodide
• Saturated solution
^{131}I

30 CHAPTER

Thyroid Hormones and Thyroid Inhibitors

THYROID AGONIST

- I-Thyroxine sod
- Triiodothyronine

  Uses:
  - Cretinism
  - Hypothyroidism
  - Myxedema coma
  - Nontoxic goiter
  - Thyroid nodule
  - Papillary Ca of thyroid

THYROID INHIBITORS

Inhibit Hormone Synthesis

- Propylthiouracil
- Carbimazole

  MOA: – Inhibit thyroid peroxidase enzyme

  Uses: – To control thyrotoxicosis
  – Propylthiouracil—thyrotoxicosis in pregnancy

A/E: – Fever, joint pain, agranulocytosis hypothyroidism, goiter and loss or graying of hair

Inhibit Iodide Trapping

- Nitrate
- Thiocyanate

  MOA: Inhibition of iodide trapping

Inhibit Hormone Release

Iodine

Iodide of Na^+ and K^+

MOA: Excess iodide inhibit its own transport and interfere with iodination (Wolff-Chaikoff effect)

A/E: Acute reaction
- Swelling of lip
- Angioedema
- Fever
- Joint pain
- Thrombocytopenia

Destroy Thyroid Tissue

Radioactive iodine (I^{131}, ^{125}I, ^{123}I)

Uses:
- Thyroid storm
- Preoperative preparation
- Hyperthyroidism—thyrotoxicosis, Grave's disease.

Differences Between Propylthiouracil and Carbimazole

• Less potent	• More potent
• Less duration of action	• More duration of action
• High protein bound	• Less bound
• Not cross placenta	• Cross placenta
• Inhibits peripheral conversion of T4-T3	• Does not inhibit T4-T3

DOC for hypothyroidism—thyroxine
DOC for hyperthyroidism and thyroid storm—propylthiouracil
DOC for reducing thyroid vascularity and make patient euthyroid before surgery—potassium iodide
DOC for suppressing the manifestation of hyperthyroidism—propranolol.

31 CHAPTER

Insulin and Oral Hypoglycemic Agents

INSULIN

Ultrashort acting	Insulin lispro Insulin aspart Insulin glulisine
Indications	Type I diabetes mellitus Diabetic ketoacidosis Non-ketotic hyper glycemic coma Diabetes during pregnancy
Short-term acting	Crystalline insulin
Intermediate	Isophane insulin
Long-acting	Insulin glargine Insulin detemir
Complications/side effects	Blurred vision Hypoglycemia Loss of fine motor activity Confusion Tremor Palpitation

Lipodystrophy
Insulin resistance

Edema due to salt and water retention

DOC for diabetic neuropathy—topiramate

ORAL HYPOGLYCEMIC DRUGS

Sulfonylureas

1st Generation:	Tolbutamide Chlorpropamide
2nd Generation:	Glibenclamide Glipizide Glimepiride
MOA:	Block ATP sensitive K+ channel depolarization Degranulation and release of stored insulin from pancreatic β-cell membrane
S/E:	Hypoglycemia Paresthesia Weight gain

Biguanides

Metformin **(Mr. Met)**; **(Glysiss M:** Gliclazide 80 mg + Metformin 500 mg**)**

MOA:	Inhibits hepatic gluconeogenesis Inhibits absorption from GIT Increases peripheral utilization
A/E:	Lactic acidosis Vit B_{12} deficiency

Meglitinide

- Repaglinide
- Nateglinide

MOA:	Same as biguanides
A/E:	Dyspepsia Arthralgia Weight gain

Thiazolidinediones

- Rosiglitazone
- Pioglitazone

MOA:	Agonist for PPAR Which enhances the transcription of insulin response genes
S/E:	Myalgia, weight gain, anemia, edema

α-Glucosidase Inhibitors

- Acarbose
- Miglitol

MOA:	Inhibit α-glucosidase Which is the final step in CHO metabolism
S/E:	Flatulence Fullness Diarrhea

Indication: Type II DM

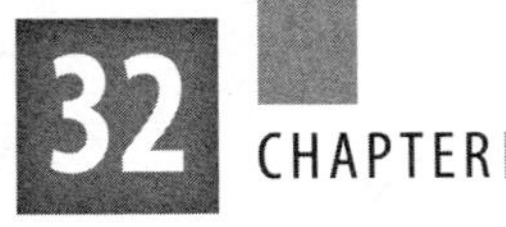

Corticosteroids

CLASSIFICATION

Short-acting	Hydrocortisone
	Cortisone
Intermediate-acting	Prednisolone
	Methylprednisolone
	Triamcinolone
Long-acting	Betamethasone
	Dexamethasone
Local-acting /Inhalational	Beclomethasone
	Budesonide
	Fluticasone

MOA: Steroid enter into cells of target organ

↓

Bind to specific receptor in cytoplasm

↓

Steroid receptor complex become activated

↓

Enter into nucleus

↓

Bind to specific site on DNA
↓
Regulate protein synthesis
↓
Response

USES OF CORTICOSTEROIDS

CORTICOSTEROIDS
Collagen disease
Osteoarthritis
Rheumatoid arthritis
Thyroid storm
Intestinal disease (ulcerative colitis and Crohn's disease)
Cerebral oedema
Organ transplantation
Skin disease
To test adrenal pituitary axis function
Eye diseases
Rheumatic fever
Other lung diseases, asthma
Infective **D**isease
Septic shock

CORTICOSTEROID SIDE EFFECTS

CUSHINGS BAD MD
Cataract
Up all right (sleep disturbance)
Suppression of HPA axis

Hypertension, buffalo **H**ump
Infection
Necrosis (avascular)
Striae
Bone loss (osteoporosis)
Acne
Diabetes
Myopathy, **M**oon faces
Depression

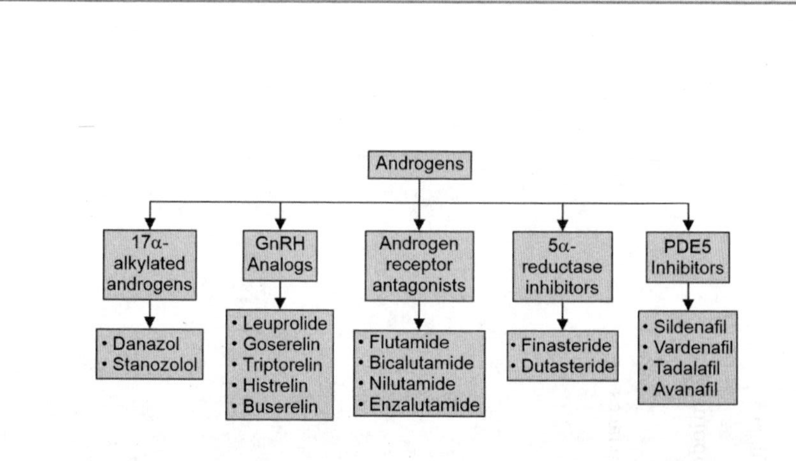

Androgens
17α-alkylated androgens
• Danazol
• Stanozolol
GnRH Analogs
• Leuprolide
• Goserelin
• Triptorelin
• Histrelin
• Buserelin
Androgen receptor antagonists
• Flutamide
• Bicalutamide
• Nilutamide
• Enzalutamide
5α-reductase inhibitors
• Finasteride
• Dutasteride
PDE5 Inhibitors
• Sildenafil
• Vardenafil
• Tadalafil
• Avanafil

33 CHAPTER

Androgens

NATURAL ANDROGENS

- Testosterone
- Dihydrotestosterone

SYNTHETIC ANDROGENS

- Methyltestosterone
- Fluoxymesterone

Uses:	– Replacement therapy in hypogonadism
	– Carcinoma of breast
	– Senile osteoporosis in men
A/E:	– In females hirsutism, breast atrophy in children
	– Impairment of growth
	– Edema
	– Cholestatic jaundice—methyltestosterone
	– Acnes
	– Gynecomastia

ANABOLIC STEROIDS

	NOSE
	Nandrolone
	Oxandrolone
	Stanozolol
	Ethylestrenol
Uses:	In chronic illness to improve appetite
	To counteract catabolic effect
	In postmenopausal and senile osteoporosis
	In chronic itching in biliary obstruction
A/E:	– Hirsutism
	– Oedema
	– Acne
	– Growth retardation
	– Gynecomastia

ANTIANDROGEN

a. Physiological	Estrogen
MOA:	Inhibiting gonadotropin secretion
b. Synthesis inhibitor	Ketoconazole—antifungal
	spironolactone
c. Receptor antagonist	Flutamide
	Cyproterone acetate
d. 5 α reductase inhibitor	Finasteride, dutasteride
MOA:	Inhibit 5 α reductase
	dihydrotestosterone
Use:	In BPH

S/E: Impotence
Rashes and itching
Decreased libido

Drugs for Erectile Dysfunction

- Sildenafil
- Tadalafil
- Vardenafil

DOC for spinal cord injury induced sexual impotence—alprostadil
DOC for BPH—tamsulosin, finasteride
DOC for oligospermia, polycystic ovarian disease—clomiphene citrate
DOC for gynecomastia, fibrocystic breast disease—danazol

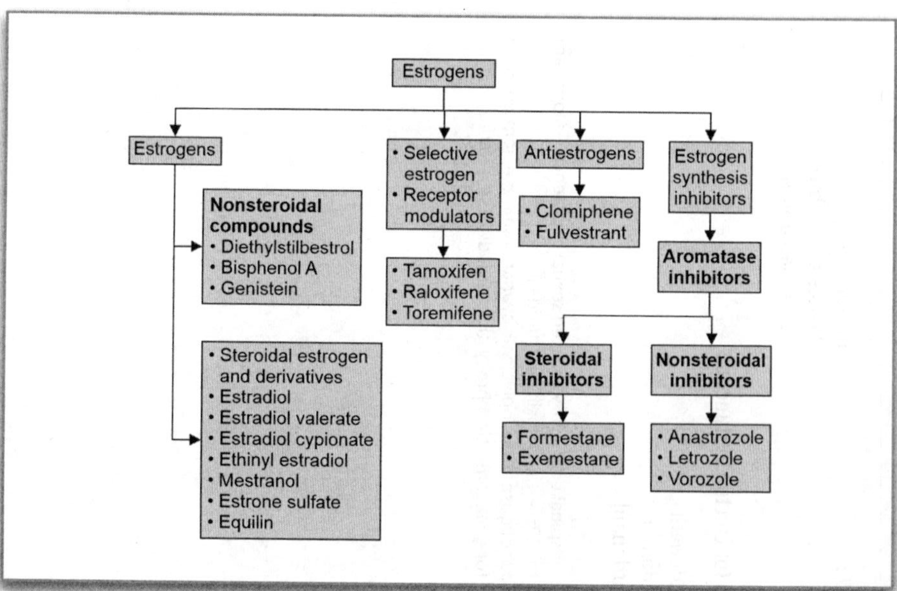
Estrogens
Estrogens
Nonsteroidal compounds
• Diethylstilbestrol
• Bisphenol A
• Genistein
• Steroidal estrogen and derivatives
• Estradiol
• Estradiol valerate
• Estradiol cypionate
• Ethinyl estradiol
• Mestranol
• Estrone sulfate
• Equilin
• Selective estrogen
• Receptor modulators
• Tamoxifen
• Raloxifene
• Toremifene
Antiestrogens
• Clomiphene
• Fulvestrant
Estrogen synthesis inhibitors
Aromatase inhibitors
Steroidal inhibitors
• Formestane
• Exemestane
Nonsteroidal inhibitors
• Anastrozole
• Letrozole
• Vorozole

34 CHAPTER

Estrogens

ESTROGEN

Natural	Estradiol, estriol
Synthetic-steroidal	Ethinyl estradiol
Nonsteroidal	Diethyl estradiol
Uses:	Oral contraceptive
	Carcinoma prostate
	Dysmenorrhea
	Delayed puberty
A/E:	Breast tenderness
	Carcinoma of endometrium
	Carcinoma of breast
	Oedema

ANTIESTROGEN

- Clomiphene citrate
- Fulvestrant

MOA: Competitively block estrogen receptor in anterior pituitary

↓

Inhibit negative feedback of estrogen
↓
Release of gonadotropin
↓
Induce ovulation

Uses:	In fertility—due to anovulation
	In vitro fertilization
	Male infertility
A/E:	Multiple pregnancy
	Ovarian malignancy
	Ovarian cyst

Selective Estrogen Receptor Modulators (SERMs)

Tamoxifen	*Uses:* Ca breast; *A/E:* Edema, endometrial carcinoma, DVT
Raloxifene	*Uses:* Treatment of osteoporosis, *A/E:* Leg cramps, DVT

PROGESTIN

Natural	Progesterone **(Gestmate)**
Derivatives	Megestrol acetate

19-Nortestosterone Derivatives

- Norethindrone
- Levonorgestrel

Uses:

- Contraception
- HRT in postmenopausal females
- Endometriosis

- Carcinoma of endometrium
- Postponing the periods

A/E:
- Acne
- Oedema
- Thromboembolism
- Weight gain

ANTIPROGESTIN

Mifepristone

MOA: Competitively antagonist of progesterone has luteolytic property

Uses:
- Termination of pregnancy
- Contraception
- Induction of labor
- Cervical ripening
- Cushing's syndrome—mifepristone has palliative effect

A/E:
- Abdominal discomfort
- Uterine bleeding
- Teratogenicity

DOC for prevention of breast cancer—tamoxifen.

35 CHAPTER

Drugs Acting on Uterus

CLASSIFICATION

Uterine Stimulant

Oxytocin **E**xcites **P**regnant **U**terus

- **O**xytocin
- **E**rgometrine
- **P**rostaglandins—PGE_2, PGF_2, Misoprostol

MOA:
- G-Coupled oxytocin receptor
- Depolarization and influx of calcium
- Contraction of uterus

Uses:
- Induction labor
- PPH
- Breast engorgement

Uterine Relaxant

- **Mg B**lock **C**ontraction **Of P**regnant uterus
- **Mg** sulphate
- β_2- agonist—**FIRST**

Fenoterol
Isoxsuprine
Ritodrine
Salbutamol
Terbutaline

Calcium-channel blocker: Nifedipine
Oxytocin antagonist: Atosiban
PG synthesis inhibitors: Aspirin
Ibuprofen
NSAID

DOC for priming or ripening of cervix—dinoprost
DOC for inducing labor—oxytocin

36 CHAPTER

Drugs Affecting Calcium Balance

CALCIUM

Oral	Calcium orotate (orotate)
	Calcium gluconate
	Calcium citrate
	Calcium carbonate
Parenteral	IV calcium gluconate
	IV calcium chloride
Uses:	To correct calcium deficiency
	In tetany
	Calcium carbonate—antacid
	To treat urticaria and dermatosis
	To correct osteoporosis
A/E:	Constipation
	Bloating and excess gas formation

DOC for osteoporosis—raloxifene

CALCITONIN

- Procaine calcitonin
- Salmon calcitonin

- Synthetic calcitonin

  Uses: Hypercalcemic state
  Paget's disease
  In postmenopausal osteoporosis

VITAMIN-D

Ergocalciferol	Used in rickets in children's, osteomalacia in adult
Cholecalciferol	
Calcitriol	Postmenopausal osteoporosis
Alfacalcidol	Effective in renal bone disease and hypoparathyroidism
Calcipotriol	Topical use in psoriasis

BISPHOSPHONATES

1st generation	Etidronate
2nd generation	– Pamidronate
	– Alendronate
3rd generation	– Risedronate
	– Zoledronate

MOA:

Antiresorptive effect

↓

High affinity for calcium in bone

↓

Accumulate in area of resorption

↓

Taken up by osteoclast

↓

Promote their apoptosis

Uses:

- Paget's disease
- Postmenopausal osteoporosis
- In hypercalcemia of malignancy
- To relieve pain of lytic bone lesion

A/E:

- Hypocalcemia
- Esophagitis in oral treatment
- Flu-like symptoms in parenteral treatment

DOSAGE OF HORMONES AND RELATED DRUGS

Somatropin	0.03–0.07 mg/kg—in pituitary dwarfism
	0.05–0.1 mg/kg—in AIDS related wasting
Somatostatin	250 μg slowly IV over 3 min
Octreotide	50–100 μg SC twice daily up to 500 μg TDS
	100 μg IV esophageal variceal bleeding
Bromocriptine	2.5–1 mg BD—hyperprolactinemia
	5–20 mg /day—acromegaly
Cabergoline	Start with 0.25 mg twice weekly, up to 1 mg
Nafarelin	400 μg BD intranasal } assisted reproduction
	200 μg BD when menstrual bleeding
	200 μg BD for 3–6 months—uterine fibroids
	200 μg BD up to 6 months—endometriosis
	800 μg BD by nasal spray—central precocious puberty
Triptorelin	2.5–3.5 mg IM at 3–4 weeks interval
L-Thyroxine sodium	8–12 μg/kg/day—cretinism
	50 μg daily up to 100–200 μg/day—A/C hypothyroidism
	200–500 μg IV then 100 μg IV OD—myxedema coma
Propylthiouracil	50–150 mg TDS then 25–50 mg BD
Methimazole	5–10 mg TDS
Carbimazole	5–15 mg TDS
Iodide	100–300 mg/day—therapeutic
	5–10 mg/day—prophylactic

Tolbutamide	0.5–3 g/day
Chlorpropamide	0.1–0.5 g/day
Glibenclamide	1–2 mg/day
Glipizide	5–20 mg
Glimepiride	1–6 mg/day
Metformin	0.5–2.5 g
Repaglinide	1.5–8 mg
Rosiglitazone	4–8 mg
Pioglitazone	14–45 mg
Hydrocortisone	20 mg morning + 10 afternoon orally 100 mg IV bolus + 100 mg 8 hourly IV infusion—shock, status asthmaticus, A/C renal insufficiency
Prednisolone	5–60 mg/day oral
Methylprednisolone	4–32 mg/day oral
Triamcinolone	4–32 mg
Dexamethasone	0.5–5 mg/day oral
Betamethasone	0.5–5 mg/day oral, 4–20 mg IM, IV—cerebral edema
Fludrocortisone	50–200 μg /daily-Addison's disease 100–200 μg/daily idiopathic postural hypotension
Testosterone	25 mg IM daily
Testosterone propionate	25–50 mg daily
Methandienone	2–5 mg OD-BD oral
Nandrolone	10–50 mg IM once weekly

Oxymetholone	5–10 mg OD
Stanozolol	2–6 mg/day
Danazol	200–600 mg/day
Finasteride	5 mg OD—BPH 1 mg/daily—male pattern of baldness
Dutasteride	0.5 mg OD—BPH, Ca prostate, baldness
Sildenafil	50 mg, if not effective 100 mg 1 hour before intercourse
Tadalafil	10 mg at least 30 min before intercourse
Estradiol	2.5–10 mg IM
Ethinylestradiol	0.02–0.2 mg/day oral
Tibolone	2.5 mg daily
Clomiphene citrate	50 mg OD
Tamoxifen citrate	10–20 mg BD
Raloxifene	60 mg/day
Ormeloxifen	120 mg twice weekly
Letrozole	2.5 mg BD oral
Anastrozole	1 mg OD oral
Progesterone	10–100 mg IM OD
Mifepristone	Single 400 mg oral—complete abortion followed by 400 mg oral after 48 hour 600 mg 1–2 days before labor—cervical ripening 600 mg given with in 72 hours—postcoital contraceptives
Oxytocin (1 IU = 2 μg)	5 IU diluted in 500 mL of glucose-Induction of labor

	5 IU IM/IV—PPH
	25–50 IV just before breastfeeding—breast engorgement
Ergometrine	0.2–0.3 mg IM at delivery of anterior shoulder
	0.5 mg IV, if PPH started
Ritodrine	10 mg IV/IM
Nifedipine	10 mg every 20–30 min till contraction stop
Magnesium sulfate	2–4 g IV bolus over 10–20 min then 1 g hourly
Calcium	10–20 mL of calcium gluconate
Calcitonin	4–8 IU/kg IM 6–12 hourly—hyperparathyroidism
	100 IU SC/IM daily—postmenopausal osteoporosis
	100 IU daily on alternative days—Paget's disease

10 SECTION

Drugs Affecting Blood

- Hypolipidemic Drugs
- Plasma Expanders

37 CHAPTER

Hypolipidemic Drugs

STATINS

PARSAL
Pravastatin
Atorvastatin
Rosuvastatin
Simvastatin
Atorvastatin
Lovastatin

MOA:	Inhibit HMG-CoA reductase (rate-limiting enzyme)
A/E:	**MESS** **M**yopathy **E**levation of liver transaminase **S**leep disturbance **S**evere hepatotoxicity

BILE ACID SEQUESTRANTS (RESINS)

- Cholestyramine
- Colestipol

MOA: Decrease bile acid absorption

↓

Increase hepatic conversion of cholesterol to bile acid

↓

Increase LDL receptor on hepatocyte

A/E: **TFC**

Increased **T**G level

Flatulence

Constipation

FIBRIC ACID DERIVATIVES

BC de **FG**

Bezafibrate

Clofibrate

Fenofibrate

Gemfibrozil

MOA: Increase activity of lipoprotein lipase

↓

Decrease release of fatty acid from adipose tissue

NICOTINIC ACID

Best drug to increase HDL

MOA: Decrease production of VLDL

↓

Decrease lipolysis in adipocyte

OTHERS

- Ezetimibe
- Gugulipid

DOC for LDL cholesterol reduction—HMG-COA reductase
DOC for increasing HDL cholesterol—niacin
DOC for reducing TAG Level—fibrates

38 CHAPTER

Plasma Expanders

CLASSIFICATION

- Dextran 40, 70
- Human albumin
- Hydroxyethyl starch (HES)
- Polyvinyl pyrrolidone

Uses:	Burns
	Hypovolemic shock
	Trauma
C/I:	Cardiac failure
	Pulmonary edema
	Renal failure
	Anemia

IDEAL PLASMA EXPANDER

- Should not be antigenic and pyrogenic
- Pharmacologically inert
- Should exert oncotic pressure comparable to plasma
- Should remain in circulation and not leak out in tissue or be too rapidly disposed
- Should be stable

Crystalloids

- Dextrose
- DNS and RL

  Uses: Diarrhea
  Vomiting
  Water loss in diabetes insipidus
  Renal impairment and heat stroke

11 SECTION

Antimicrobial Drugs

39 CHAPTER

Sulfonamides and Cotrimoxazole

SULFONAMIDES

Bacteriostatic

C/S:		
–	Short acting (4–8 hours)	Sulfadiazine
–	Intermediate acting (8–12 hours)	Sulfamethoxazole
–	Long acting (up to 7 days)	Sulfadoxine
–	Special purpose sulfonamide	Mafenide
		Silver sulfadiazine
		Sulfasalazine

MOA: PABA
↓ Inhibit bacterial folate synthesis
DHFA
↓
DNA synthesis

SIDE EFFECTS OF SULFONAMIDES

SULFONAMIDES
Stevens-Johnson syndrome
Urticaria
Leukopenia

Photosensitivity
Hemolytic Anemia + Hepatitis
Obstruction of urinary tract
Nausea
Agranulocytosis
Malaise, **M**egaloblastic anemia
Increased risk of kernicterus in newborn
Depression, **D**rug fever
Eosinophilia
Skin rashes

Uses:
- UTI (Suppressive therapy)
- Toxoplasmosis
- Trachoma (ocular sulfacetamide. sod)
- Nocardia
- Malaria

COTRIMOXAZOLE

Sulfamethoxazole + Trimethoprim (5:1)

MOA: Sequential inhibition

PABA
↓
DHFA
↓
THFA

Uses:
- UTI
- RTI
- Bacterial gastroenteritis
- Typhoid
- Chancroid

A/E:
- Glossitis
- Stomatitis
- May PPT megaloblastic anemia
- Uremia in renal patient
- Should be avoided in pregnancy

40 CHAPTER

Quinolones and Fluoroquinolones

QUINOLONES

NOC
Nalidixic acid
Oxalinic acid
Cinoxacin

MOA:	–	Inhibit DNA gyrase
Uses:	–	UTI—*E. coli, Proteus*
	–	Diarrhea—*Shigella*
A/E:	–	Vertigo
	–	Biliary stasis
	–	Hemolysis
	–	Leukopenia

FLUOROQUINOLONE

First generation

CON P
Ciprofloxacin
Ofloxacin
Norfloxacin
Pefloxacin

Second generation	Lomefloxacin Levofloxacin Sparfloxacin Gemifloxacin Moxifloxacin
MOA:	Inhibit DNA gyrase Inhibit topoisomerase 4
Uses:	UTI-Norfloxacin 400 mg BD Typhoid—ciprofloxacin 500 mg BD Gonorrhea Chancroid RTI

CIPROFLOXACIN

- Prototype, 1st given drug
- *Spectrum:* Aerobic gram-negative bacteria

Highly susceptible

- *E. Coli*
- *N. gonorrhoeae,* meningitidis
- *H. influenzae*
- *Salmonella typhi*
- *Vibrio cholerae*

Four remarkable microbiological properties:

1. Rapid bactericidal activity + increase potency
2. Long postantibiotic effect
3. Low frequency of resistance
4. Protective intestinal streptococci are spared.

A/E: **RATT**
Reversible arthritis
Arthropathy
Tendosynovitis
Tendon rupture

C/I: In pregnancy

41 CHAPTER

Beta-lactam Antibiotics

PENICILLIN

Natural: Penicillin G
(Benzyl penicillin)

Uses:

- Streptococcal infection
- Pneumococcal infection
- Meningococcal infection, tetanus, gas gangrene
- Gonorrhea, syphilis, diphtheria

Acid Resistant Penicillin

Penicillin v—*Neisseria*

Penicillinase Resistant Penicillins

- Methicillin
- Cloxacillin—for staphylococci except MRSA

Extended Spectrum

- Aminopenicillin
  - Ampicillin
  - Amoxicillin — All organs sensitive to penicillin+ *H. influenzae* *E. coli* *Proteus, Shigella, Salmonella*
- Carboxypenicillin
  - Carbenicillin
  - Ticarcillin — Against *Pseudomonas* and *Proteus*
- Ureidopenicillin
  - Piperacillin
  - Mezlocillin—*Klebsiella*

MOA: Penicillin—inhibit cell wall synthesis

↓

Penicillin bind to PBP (penicillin-binding protein)

↓

Inhibit cross-linking of peptide

↓

Cell wall deficient bacteria

↓

Lysis

↓

Bactericidal effect

A/E:

- Local—thrombophlebitis of injected vein
- Hypersensitivity
  - » Anaphylaxis
  - » Angioedema
  - » Bronchospasm
  - » Jarisch Herxheimer reaction

β-lactamase Inhibitor

- Clavulanic acid
- Sulbactam
- Tazobactam

MOA: Inhibition of β-lactamase enzyme—suicidal inhibition

Spectrum:
- *Staph. aureus*
- *H. influenzae*
- *N. gonorrhoeae*
- *E. coli*
- *Proteus*
- *Klebsiella, Salmonella, Shigella*

A/E: *Candida stomatitis*
Vaginitis

42 CHAPTER

Cephalosporins

CLASSIFICATION

Generation	*Parenteral*	*Oral*
First generation	Cefazolin	Cephalexin Cefadroxil
Second generation	Cefuroxime	Cefuroxime axetil Cefaclor
Third generation	Ceftriaxone Cefotaxime	Cefixime Cefpodoxime proxetil
Fourth generation	Cefepime Cefpirome	

MOA: Inhibit bacterial cell wall synthesis

A/E:
- Pain at site of injection
- Diarrhea
- Nephrotoxicity
- Bleeding
- Neutropenia and thrombocytopenia
- Disulfiram like reaction

Uses:
- Enteric fever
- Alternative to penicillin
- RTI, UTI, by gram positive bacteria
- Septicemia
- Meningitis
- Gonorrhea

43 CHAPTER

Tetracyclines and Chloramphenicol

TETRACYCLINES

Bacteriostatic

MOA:	Inhibits attachment of aminoacyl tRNA to A site of 30s ribosome
Uses:	**"C" VARRP** **C**holera **V**enereal disease **A**typical pneumonia **R**ickettsia **R**elapsing fever **P**lague
Side effects:	**DISH*** **D**ose related—hepato-, nephro-, phototoxicity **I**rritative **S**uperinfection **H**ypersensitivity—urticaria, angioedema

CHLORAMPHENICOL

MOA: Inhibits bacterial protein synthesis by interfering with transfer of elongating peptide chain to the newly attached amino-acyl tRNA at ribosome mRNA complex

Uses:
- Enteric fever, bacterial meningitis
- Anaerobic infection
- Intraocular infection
- UTI

A/E:
- ***ISH** + Gray baby syndrome
- Bone marrow depression

44 CHAPTER

Aminoglycoside Antibiotics

SYSTEMIC

- Streptomycin
- Gentamicin
- Kanamycin
- Tobramycin
- Amikacin

TOPICAL

- Neomycin
- Framycetin

MOA:

AG (Aminoglycoside)
↓
Penetrate cell membrane
↓
Reach periplasmic space
↓
Bind to 30s ribosome
↓
Inhibit protein synthesis
↓
Bactericidal

General spectrum: Aerobic Gram negative bacilli

Uses:
- Gram negative bacteria
- Streptococcal
- Enterococcal
- Tuberculosis—streptomycin
- *Pseudomonas* and *Proteus*—tobramycin, amikacin
- Meningitis

A/E:
- Ototoxicity
- Nephrotoxicity
- Neuromuscular blockade
- Superinfection

45 CHAPTER

Macrolide Antibiotics

CLASSIFICATION

CARE

Clarithromycin: Triple regimen of *H. pylori*
Azithromycin
Roxithromycin
Erythromycin

MOA:

Inhibit bacterial protein synthesis
↓
By binding with 50s ribosome
↓
Inhibit translocation of peptide chain
↓
Inhibit cell wall synthesis

Uses: Remember National Immunization Schedule
DPT Measles, **P**olio and **BCG**
Diphtheria
Pertussis
Tetanus, ***T**oxoplasma gondii*
***M**ycoplsma*

Atypical **P**neumonia
***B**acterial diarrhea*
Chancroid
***G**enital infection*

A/E:

Hepatitis + Cholestatic jaundice
Reversible hearing loss
Cardiac arrhythmias

CLINDAMYCIN

MOA:

Bind to 50s ribosomal unit
↓
Suppress protein synthesis
↓
Inhibit bacterial multiplication

Spectrum

- *Streptococcus*
- *Staphylococcus*
- Pneumococci
- *Toxoplasma gondii*
- *Bact. fragilis*

A/E:
- Diarrhea
- *Pseudomembranous colitis*

VANCOMYCIN

MOA: Bind to peptidoglycan chain
↓
Inhibit elongation of protein chain
↓
Weak cell wall
↓
Bacterial lysis

Uses: Orally for pseudomembranous colitis and MRSA

A/E: **Red man syndrome:** Rapid IV injection has caused chills, fever, urticaria and severe flushing
Ototoxicity
Nephrotoxicity

46 CHAPTER

Antitubercular Drugs

1st line drugs	*MOA*	*A/E: Hepatotoxicity in all drugs*
Isoniazid—**INH**	• Inhibit mycolic acid synthesis • Effective against both intra and extracellular—tuberculocidal	**I**nsanity, **N**euritis, **H**epatitis
RIFampicin	• Inhibit DNA dependent RNA polymerase—tuberculocidal • Effective against intra- and extracellular including spurters	**R**eddish orange urine **I**nduction of liver enzyme **F**lu-like syndrome
Pyrazinamide	• Inhibit mycolic acid synthesis • Effective against intracellular bacilli—Bactericidal • Bacteriostatic drug	**P**ain in joint **P**lus hepatitis (hyperuricemia and gout)

Contd...

Contd...

Streptomycin—**NON**	Inhibit protein synthesis	Similar to AG **N**eurotoxicity
	Effective against extracellular bacilli—Bactericidal	**O**totoxicity **N**ephrotoxicity
Ethambutol	• Inhibit arabinosyl-transferase	**E**ye toxicity Optic neuritis Color blindness

Dosage of antitubercular drugs—**PESRI**

Pyrazinamide (z): 25 mg/kg
Ethambutol: 15 mg/kg
Streptomycin: 15 mg/kg
Rifampicin: 10 mg/kg
Isoniazid (H): 5 mg/kg

DOTS Regime (Directly observed treatment short course):

Category 1: New patients

- *Intensive phase:* 2 $H_3 R_3 Z_3 E_3$ (2-two months, 3-thrice weekly)
- *Continuation phase:* 4 $H_3 R_3$

Category 2: Previously treated patients

- *Intensive phase:* 2 $H_3 R_3 Z_3 E_3 S_3$ + 1 $H_3 R_3 Z_3 E_3$
- *Continuation phase:* 5 $H_3 R_3 E_3$

2nd line drugs

Ciprofloxacin	Para-aminosalicylic acid
Kanamycin	Rifabutin
Cycloserin	Ethionamide
Amikacin	Thiacetazone

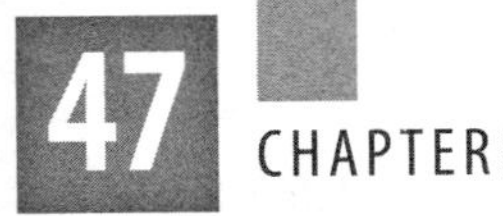

Antileprotic Drugs

CLASSIFICATION

Sulfone	Dapsone
Phenazine derivative	Clofazimine
Antitubercular drugs	Rifampin Ethionamide
Other antibiotics	Ofloxacin
	Minocycline
	Clarithromycin
	Moxifloxacin

DAPSONE

MOA: Inhibit incorporation of PABA into folic acid

Uses:
- Leprosy
- Chloroquine-resistant malaria along with pyrimethamine

A/E:
- Hemolytic anemia in G6PD deficiency
- Methemoglobinemia

CLOFAZIMINE

MOA: Block function of DNA
A/E: Reddish black discoloration of skin

48 CHAPTER

Antifungal Drugs

CLASSIFICATION

a. Antibiotics — Amphotericin B, nystatin
Hamycin, griseofulvin

b. Antimetabolites — Flucytosine

c. Azoles

Imidazole	*Triazoles*
• Econazole	• Fluconazole
• Miconazole	• Itraconazole
• Ketoconazole	
• Clotrimazole	

d. Topical agents — Benzoic acid, salicylic acid

AMPHOTERICIN B

MOA: Amphotericin B bind to ergosterol
↓
Make pore in the cell membrane
↓
Cell content leak out

Spectrum:
- *Candida, Histoplasma*
- *Cryptococcus, Aspergillus*

A/E:
- Renal tubular acidosis
- Nephrotoxicity
- Anemia

GRISEOFULVIN

MOA:
- Griseofulvin bind to microtubular protein
- Deposited in skin protection from new infection inhibit mitosis

Uses: Superficial dermatophytosis

A/E:
- Hepatitis
- Neurotoxicity

FLUCYTOSINE

MOA: Inhibit DNA synthesis

Uses: Along with amphotericin B and azole

A/E: BM depression

AZOLES

MOA: Inhibit fungal cytochrome enzyme Lanosterol-14-demethylase

↓

Impair ergosterol synthesis

↓

Defective cell membrane/membrane abnormality in fungus

Uses:	Candidiasis Dermatophytosis Cryptococcal meningitis Coccidioidal meningitis
A/E:	Hepatotoxicity Gynecomastia Lose of libido Menstrual irregularities

49 CHAPTER

Anthelmintic Drugs

CLASSIFICATION

- *For roundworm, hookworm and pinworm:* Albendazole, mebendazole, pyrantel pamoate, piperazine
- *For whipworm and Trichinella spiralis:* Albendazole, mebendazole
- *For tapeworms:* Praziquantel, albendazole
- *Hydatid disease:* Albendazole, mebendazole
- *For thread worm:* Ivermectin, albendazole
- *For filariasis:* Diethylcarbamazine, ivermectin, albendazole

MOA: Bind to B tubulin
↓
Inhibit synthesis of microtubule
↓
Inhibit metabolic process

Uses: Against
Roundworm
Hookworm
Pinworm
Neurocysticercosis—albendazole
Hydatid disease
Filariasis

A/E: Alopecia
Granulocytopenia
Jaundice

Drugs for Kala-azar

KAPA Azar
Ketoconazole
Antimonial—sodium stibogluconate
Pentamidine
Amphotericin B
Allopurinol

Drugs for *Pneumocystis Carinii*

Pentamidine
Cotrimoxazole

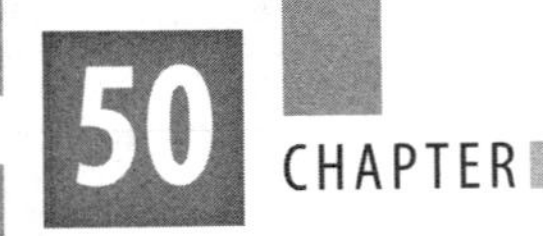

Antiamoebic Drugs

CLASSIFICATION

Intestinal	• Diloxanide furoate, iodocuinol
	• Tetracycline, paromomycin
Extraintestinal	Chloroquine
Both intestinal and extraintestinal	• Metronidazole
	• Tinidazole
	• Emetine
	• Dehydroemetine

MOA: Metronidazole
↓
Bind to DNA
↓
Inhibit protein synthesis

Uses: **H GATE**
H. *pylori*
Giardiasis
Amoebiasis
T*richomonas*
E*ntamoeba*

A/E:
- Metallic taste
- Peripheral neuritis
- Stomatitis
- Glossitis

C/I: Metronidazole produces disulfiram-like reaction. So they should be instructed to avoid drinking.

51 CHAPTER

Antimalarial Drugs

CLASSIFICATION

Causal prophylaxis:	• Proguanil	
	• Primaquine: Tissue schizonticide	
Clinical and suppressive cure:	• Chloroquine	• Pyrimethamine
	• Quinine	• Proguanil
	• Mefloquine	• Sulfadoxine
	• Atovaquone	• Doxycycline
	• Artesunate	
Radical cure (hypnoidal):	Primaquine	
Gametocidal drugs:	Primaquine	
	Quinine	

CHLOROQUINE

MOA: Chloroquine—It concentrate in infected RBC mainly in vesicles of parasite and inhibit conversion of heme to hemozoin by forming heme-chloroquine complex—this complex toxic and kill the parasite.

Other uses: **MALARIA**

- **M**alaria
- **A**moebiasis
- **L**epra reaction
- **R**heumatoid **A**rthritis
- **I**nfectious mononucleosis
- **A**utoimmune disorders (DLC)

A/E:

- Irreversible retinopathy
- Neuropathy
- Myopathy
- Cardiomyopathy

QUININE AND QUINIDINE

MOA: Same as chloroquine

Uses:

- Cerebral malaria
- Chloroquine resistant malaria
- Nocturnal leg cramps

A/E:

- Cinchonism
- Black water fever
- Hypotension
- Hypoglycemia

52 CHAPTER

Antiviral Drugs

CLASSIFICATION

Antiherpes Virus

- Acyclovir
- Valacyclovir
- Famciclovir

Antiretrovirus

Nucleoside reverse transcriptase inhibitor (NRTI)
- Zidovudine
- Stavudine
- Lamivudine
- Abacavir

Non-nucleoside reverse transcriptase inhibitor
- Nevirapine
- Efavirenz

Protease inhibitors
- Ritonavir
- Nelfinavir
- Lopinavir

- Saquinavir
- Indinavir

Anti-influenza Virus

AROZ

Amantadine
Rimantadine
Oseltamivir
Zanamivir

Nonselective Antiviral Drugs

- Ribavirin, lamivudine
- Adefovir, dipivoxil
- Interferon-alpha

MOA: Acyclovir
↓
Acyclovir triphosphate
↓
Inhibit viral DNA synthesis and viral replication

A/E:
- Neurotoxicity
- Burning sensation

MOA: Antiretrovirus
Viral RNA
↓ Inhibit this step
Viral DNA
↓
Integrate with host DNA

Viral mRNA
↓
Viral proteins
↓
Budding, release and maturation

A/E:
- BM suppression
- Long use—hepatotoxicity
- Myopathy
- Lactic acidosis

MOA:
- Anti-influenza
- Prevent viral replication

A/E:
- Teratogenicity
- Hallucination and hypotension

DOSAGE OF ANTIBIOTICS

Sulfadiazine	0.5 g QID to 2 g TDS
Sulfamethoxazole	1 g BD for 2 days, then 0.5 g BD
Cotrimoxazole (1 : 5)	Trimethoprime 80 mg + Sulfamethoxazole 400 mg; 2 BD for 2 day
Nalidixic acid	0.5–1 g TDS/QID
Sodium penicillin G	0.5–5 MU IM/IV 6–12 hourly
Procaine penicillin G	0.5–1 MU IM 12–24 hourly
Benzathine penicillin	0.6–2.4 MU every 2–4 weeks
Penicillin V	250–500 mg given 6th hourly
Cloxacillin	0.25–0.5 g orally every 6 hourly
Ampicillin	0.5–2 g oral/IM/IV
Bacampicillin	400–800 mg BD
Amoxicillin	0.25–1 g IDS oral/IM
Carbenicillin	1–2 g IM or 1–5 g IV every 4–6 hourly
Piperacillin **(Akazo P)**	100–150 mg/kg/day in 3 divided doses
Clavulanic acid	0.5 g/day
Sulbactam	1–2 vial deep IM/IV
Tazobactam	0.5 combined with piperacillin 4 g IV over 30 min 8 hourly
Cefazolin	0.25 g 8 hourly (mild cases) 1 g 6 hourly (severe cases)
Cephalexin	0.25 g–1 g 6–8 hourly
Cephradine	0.25–1 g
Cefadroxil	0.5–1 g
Cefuroxime	0.75–1.5 g IM/IV 8 hourly

Cefuroxime axetil	250–500 mg BD
Cefaclor	0.25–1 g 8 hourly
Cefotaxime	1–2 g IM/IV 8 hourly
Ceftizoxime	0.5–2 g IM/IV
Ceftriaxone	Single dose of 250 mg IM
Ceftazidime	0.5–2 g IM/lV 8th hourly
Cefoperazone	1–3 g IM/lV 8–12 hourly
Cefixime	200–800 mg BD
Cefpodoxime proxetil	200 mg BD
Cefdinir	300 mg BD
Ceftibuten	200 mg BD
Cefetamet	500 mg BD–TDS
Cefepime	1–2 g
Cefpirome	1–2 g IM/IV
Tetracycline	250–500 mg QID or TDS
Oxytetracycline	250–500 mg QID or TDS
Demeclocycline	300 mg BD
Doxycycline	200 mg initially then 100–200 mg OD
Minocycline	200 mg initially then 100–200 mg OD
Chloramphenicol	250–500 mg 6th hourly
	50–75 mg/kg/day—pyogenic meningitis
Streptomycin	1 g IM BD for 7–10 days—acute infection
Gentamicin	3–5 mg/kg/day IM single/3 divided doses
Kanamycin	0.5 g im BD-TDS
Tobramycin	3–5 mg/kg/day 1–3 divided doses
Amikacin	15 mg/kg/day in 1–3 divided doses
	7.5 mg/kg/day—UTI

Netilmicin	4–6 mg/kg/day in 1–3 divided doses
Neomycin	0.25–1 g QID oral, 0.3–0.5% topical
Erythromycin	250–500 mg 6 hourly
Clarithromycin	250 mg BD for 7 days, Severe 500 mg BD
Azithromycin **(Azitsa)**	500 mg Once daily 1 hour before/2 hour after food
Clindamycin	150–300 mg QID oral, 200–600 mg IV 8 hourly
Vancomycin	125–500 mg 6th hourly
Teicoplanin	400 mg 1st day then 200 mg daily IV/IM
Linezolid	600 mg BD oral/N
Nitrofurantoin	50–100 mg TDS 5–10 days
Methanamine	1 g TDS or QID
Phenazopyridine	200–400 mg TDS
Dapsone	100 mg/day or less
Clofazimine	50–100 mg/day
Rifampin	600 mg Monthly- leprosy
Minocycline	100 mg/day
Clarithromycin	500 mg daily
Amphotericin	50–100 mg QID—intestinal moniliasis
Griseofulvin	125–250 mg QID
Clotrimazole	10 mg 3–4 times daily
Ketoconazole	200 mg OD/BD
Fluconazole	150 mg oral dose
Itraconazole	200 mg/day
Variconazole	250 mg OD
Zidovudine	300 mg BD
Didanosine	200 mg BD

Stavudine	40 mg BD
Lamivudine	100 mg OD—chronic hepatitis B
Abacavir	300 mg BD/600 mg OD
Nevirapine	200 mg/day, increases to 200 mg BD
Efavirenz	600 mg OD
Indinavir	800 mg TDS
Nelfinavir	750 mg TDS
Ritonavir	600 mg BD
Saquinavir	1200 mg TDS
Lopinavir	400 mg BD
Amantadine	100 mg BD
Ribavirin	200 mg QID
Adefovir dipivoxil	10 mg/day
Amodiaquine	25–35 mg/kg over 3 days
Mefloquine	15 mg/kg max 1 g
Metronidazole	800 mg TDS for 10 days—Amoebiasis
	400 mg TDS—giardiasis, trichomonas vaginalis
Tinidazole	2 g OD for 3 days—amoebiasis
	2 g single dose—trichomoniasis
Secnidazole	2 g single dose
Aztreonam	0.5–2 g IM/IV 6–12 hourly
Meropenem	0.5–2 g slow IV 8 hourly
Faropenem	200–300 mg oral
Acyclovir	5–15 mg/kg/day
Valacyclovir	0.5–1 g BD-TDS
Famcyclovir	250 mg–500 mg TDS/BD

12 SECTION

Chemotherapy

- Anticancer Drugs

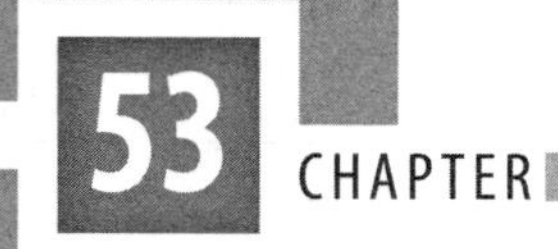

Anticancer Drugs

CYTOTOXIC AGENTS

Alkylating agents	Cyclophosphamide, mechlorethamine
	Melphalan, busulfan
Antimetabolite	Methotrexate, 6-mercaptopurine, 5-fluorouracil
Plant products	Vincristine, vinblastine
	Docetaxel, etoposide
Antibiotics	Actinomycin-D, bleomycin
	Doxorubicin, daunorubicin

DRUGS ALTERING HORMONE

Glucocorticoids	Prednisolone
SERMS	Tamoxifen, raloxifene
SERDS	Fulvestrant
5α Reductase inhibitor	Finasteride, dutasteride

CHOICE OF DRUGS

ALL	**VAMP**
	Vincristine
	Methotrexate (**A**ntimetabolite)
	6 **M**ercaptopurine
	Prednisolone
CLL	**C**hlorambucil
CML	Busulfan
Hodgkin's disease	**MOPP**
	Mechlorethamine
	Oncovin
	Prednisolone
	Procarbazine
Multiple myeloma	**M**elphalan
Ewing's sarcoma	**ADCV**
	Actinomycin
	Doxorubicin
	Cyclophosphamide
	Vincristine
Wilm's tumor	Vincristine
Breast Ca	Tamoxifen, methotrexate
Ovarian Ca	Cisplatin, carboplatin
Ca endometrium	Progestin
Testicular Ca	Methotrexate
Ca lung	Cyclophosphamide
Ca cervix	Mitomycin, methotrexate

GENERAL SIDE EFFECTS

2 Suppression	Bone marrow suppression Immunosuppression
3 **Gs**	**G**IT—stomatitis, shedding of mucosa **G**onad—oligospermia, amenorrhea, infertility **G**out
2Genicity	Teratogenicity Carcinogenicity—secondary cancer—lymphoma, leukemia
Hair	Alopecia
Skin	Dermatitis

SPECIFIC SIDE EFFECTS

Cyclophosphamide	Hemorrhagic **C**ystitis
Methotrexate	Megaloblastic anemia
Busulfan, bleomycin	Pulmonary fibrosis
Doxorubicin, daunorubicin	Cardiotoxicity
Vincristine, paclitaxel	Peripheral neuritis
Cisplatin	Renal toxicity
L-asparaginase	Pancreatitis, hepatotoxicity

13 SECTION

Miscellaneous Drugs

- Immunosuppressant Drugs
- Chelating Agents
- Mnemonics
- Adverse Effect
- Drug of Choice
- Treatment of Acute Cases
- Drug Interaction

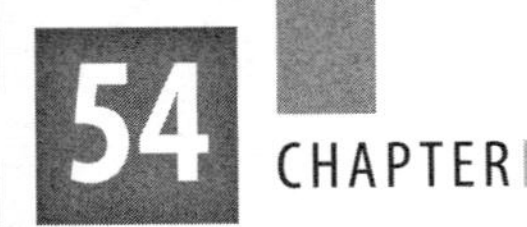

CHAPTER 54

Immunosuppressant Drugs

CLASSIFICATION

Calcineurin inhibitors	Cyclosporine, tacrolimus
Antiproliferative drugs	Azathioprine, cyclophosphamide, methotrexate, chlorambucil, mycophenolate mofetil
Glucocorticoids	Prednisolone and others
Antibodies	Muromonab CD3, antithymocyte globulin (ATG)
	Rho (D) immunoglobulin

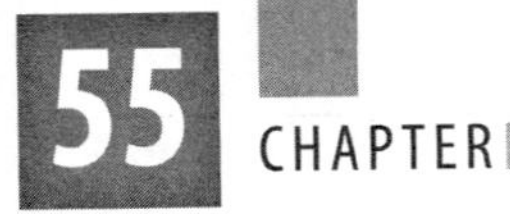

Chelating Agents

CHELATING AGENTS

These agents are classified as below:

Dimercaprol (BAL):
- Bind with As, Hg, Au, Ni, Bi, Cu
- Used as adjuvant in Cu and Pb poisoning
- Antihistamines are given to reduce tachycardia and hypotension.

Dimercaptosuccinic acid:
- Similar to BAL
- Orally active agent
- Effective against As, Hg and Pb poisoning.

Disodium EDTA:
- Chelator of calcium
- Used in emergency control of hypercalcemia
- Should be given as slow IV.
  S/E: Tetany

Calcium disodium EDTA:
- *Highly ionized compound:* Not absorbed from GIT—given IV.
- Used in lead poisoning
- Other uses are Fe, Zn, Cu, Mn and in radioactive metal poisoning.

Penicillamine

It is degradation product of penicillin. Orally absorbed

Uses:
- Wilson's disease (hepatolenticular degeneration)
- Copper and mercury poisoning
- Chronic lead poisoning
- Cystinuria and cystine stones
- Scleroderma.

Desferrioxamine

High affinity for iron—1 g is capable of chelating 85 mg of elemental iron given parenterally.

S/E: Histamine release—allergic reaction

Uses: Acute iron poisoning—most important indication

Transfusion siderosis—occurs in thalassemia patients who receive repeated blood transfusion—0.5–1 g/day IM

Deferiprone: Newer iron chelator.
Side effect and cost of treatment reduced.
Indicated in A/C iron poisoning and for in liver cirrhosis.

Thalidomide: Phocomelia, multiple defects.

Anticancer drugs (methotrexate): Cleft palate, hydrocephalus, fetal death.

Tetracycline: Discolored and deformed teeth and retarded bone growth.

Warfarin: Depressed nose, eyes and hand defects.

Phenytoin: Hydantoin syndromes.

Alcohol: Low IQ baby, growth retardation, fetal alcohol syndrome.

ACE inhibitors: Hypoplasia of organs, growth retardation, fetal loss.

Lithium: Fetal goiter, cardiac abnormality.

Indomethacin: Premature closure of ductus arteriosus.

Isotretinoin: Craniofacial, heart and CNS defect.

Chloramphenicol: Grey baby syndrome.

56 CHAPTER

Mnemonics

K^+ INCREASING AGENTS

K^+ BANK

K^+ sparing diuretic
Beta-blockers
ACEIs
NSAIDs
K^+ supplement

TERATOGENIC DRUGS

W/TERATOgenic

- **W**arfarin
- **T**halidomide
- **E**pilepsy decreasing agent—phenytoin, valproate, carbamazepine
- **R**etinoid
- **A**CE I
- **T**hird element—lithium
- **O**cps and other hormone (danazol)

GYNECOMASTIA CAUSING DRUGS

DISCOS

Digoxin
Isoniazid
Spironolactone
Cimetidine
Estrogens
Stilbestrol

CARDIOSELECTIVE BETA-BLOCKER

AMEBA

Atenolol
Metoprolol
Esmolol
Betaxolol, **B**isoprolol
Acebutolol

ANTIBIOTICS CONTRAINDICATED DURING PREGNANCY

M CAT

Metronidazole
Chloramphenicol
Aminoglycoside
Tetracyclin

DRUGS CONTRAINDICATED IN KIDNEY DISEASES

These **A**re **N**ot **P**referred in **K**idney Patients **B**ecause

Teracycline
Aminoglycoside, **A**CEI, **A**mphotericin B, **A**cyclovir

NSAID, **N**alidixic acid, **N**itrofurantoin
Phenformin
K$^+$ sparing diuretics
Penicillamine
Beta-lactam antibiotics

ANTITUBERCULOSIS DRUGS

If you forget your TB drugs you will die and might need a—**PRIEST**
Pyrazinamide
Rifampicin
Isoniazid
Ethambutol
STreptomycin

CORTICOSTEROID SIDE EFFECTS

CUSHINGS BAD MD
Cataract
Up all right (sleep disturbance)
Suppression of HPA axis
Hypertension, buffalo **H**ump
Infection
Necrosis (avascular)
Striae
Bone loss (osteoporosis)
Acne
Diabetes
Myopathy, **M**oon faces
Depression

RHEUMATIC FEVER—JONES 5 MAJOR CRITERIA

SPACE

- **S**ubcutaneous nodules
- **P**ancarditis
- **A**rthritis
- **C**horea
- **E**rythema marginatum

BETA-BLOCKER SIDE EFFECTS

BBC Losses **V**iewers **I**n **R**esia

- **B**radycardia
- **B**ronchospasm
- **C**laudication
- **L**ipids
- **V**ivid dreams—nightmares
- Negative **I**notropic action
- **R**educed sensitivity to hypoglycemia

DEPRESSION

Five drugs causing it—**PROMS**

- **P**ropranolol
- **R**eserpine
- **O**cps
- **M**ethyldopa
- **S**teroids

CALCIUM-CHANNEL BLOCKER USES

Ca^{++}MASH

Cerebral vasospasm/**C**HF
Angina
Migraine
Atrial flutter, fibrillation
Systemic **H**ypertension

ADR of Interferons

MY FAITH is NEUROTOXIC

MYelosuppression
FLu-like symptoms
Alopecia
Interstitial nephritis
Thyroiditis
Hepatotoxicity
Neurotoxic

ANTIBIOTICS CONTRAINDICATED IN PREGNANCY

SAFETY

Sulphonamide
Aminoglycoside
Fluoroquinolones
Erythromycin estolate
Tetracycline
Clindam**Y**cin

SEROTONIN SYNDROME COMPONENTS CAUSES

HARM

Hyperthermia
Automatic instability (delirium)
Rigidity
Myoclonus

PULMONARY INFILTRATION INDUCING DRUGS

GO BAN ME

Gold
Bleomycin, busulphan, BCNU
Amiodarone acyclovir, azathioprine
Nitrofurantoin
MElphalan, **ME**thotrexate
MEthysergide

ETOPOSIDE

Action, use, A/E: e**TOP**oside

MOA:	Inhibit **TOP**oisomerase—2
Uses:	**T**esticular carcinoma
	Oat cell carcinoma of lung
	Prostate carcinoma
A/E:	Affect **TOP** of your head—alopecia

ANESTHESIA

Four stages—**A**nesthesiologist **E**njoy **S** and **M**

Analgesia
Excitement

Surgical anesthesia
Medullary paralysis

NITROFURANTOIN

Major side effect—**N**itro **F**ur **A**ntoin
Neuropathy (peripheral neuropathy)
Fibrosis (pulmonary fibrosis)
Anemia (hemolytic anemia)

DRUGS CAUSING HEPATIC NECROSIS

Very **A**ngry **H**epatocytes
Valproic acid
Acetaminophen
Halothane

RESPIRATORY DEPRESSION INDUCING DRUGS

STOP breathing
Sedatives and hypnotics
Trimethoprim
Opioids
Polymyxins

TORSADES de POINTES

Drugs causing—**APACHE**
Amiodarone
Procainamide
Arsenium

Cisapride
Haloperidol
Erythromycin

ALZHEIMER'S DISEASE

AD for **MGR**

Acetyl carnitine
Donepezil
Memantine
Galantamine
Rivastigmine

ANTIHYPERTENSIVE GIVING IN PREGNANCY

3Cs

Calcium-channel blocker
Cardioselective β-blocker
Central sympatholytics—clonidine

ANTIHYPERTENSIVES USED IN EMERGENCIES

SAURAV **G**ANGULY **HELP**

Sodium nitroprusside
Glyceryltrinitrate
Hydralazine
Esmolol
Labetalol
Phentolamine

ANTILEPROTICS

CD ROME

- **C**lofazimine
- **C**larithromycin
- **D**apsone
- **R**ifampicin
- **O**floxacin
- **M**inocycline
- **E**thionamide

CARDIOSELECTIVE B-BLOCKER

AMEBA

- **A**tenolol
- **M**etoprolol
- **E**smolol
- **B**etaxolol
- **A**cebutolol

DRUGS CAUSING ACETYLATION

PC SHIP

- **P**rocainamide
- **C**lonazepam
- **S**ulfonamide
- **H**ydralazine
- **I**NH
- **P**AS (para-amino salicylic acid)

THALIDOMIDE IS USEFUL IN THE TREATMENT OF

CAKE pathologies
- **C**rohn's disease
- **A**phthous ulcer
- **K**aposi's sarcoma
- **E**rythema nodosum leprosum

Uses of TCA: **DOPAMINE**
- **D**epression
- **O**bsessive compulsive disease
- **P**hobic states
- **A**nxiety
- **M**igraine
- **I**tching
- **N**europathic pain
- **E**nuresis

XYLOCAINE NOT USED WITH ADRENALINE IN

Digital **PEN**
- **D**igits (finger and toes)
- **P**enis
- **E**ar
- **N**ose tip

TREATMENT OF METHYL ALCOHOL POISONING

Symptomatic treatment + **BEFF**
- **B**icarbonate infusion
- **E**thanol
- **F**omepizole
- **F**oliron tablets

Uses of bromocriptin—malignant **HYPHAE**

- **M**alignant neuroleptic syndrome
- **HY**perprolactinemia
- **P**arkinsonism
- **H**epatic coma
- **A**cromegaly
- **E**ngorgement of breast after delivery

MACROLIDES

CARE

- **C**larithromycin
- **A**zithromycin
- **R**oxithromycin
- **E**rythromycin

Uses of corticosteroids: **CORTICOSTEROIDS**

- **C**ollagen disease
- **O**steoarthritis
- **R**heumatoid arthritis
- **T**hyroid storm
- **I**ntestinal disease (ulcerative colitis and Crohn's disease)
- **C**erebral oedema
- **O**rgan transplantation
- **S**kin disease
- **T**o test adrenal pituitary axis function
- **E**ye diseases
- **R**heumatic fever
- **O**ther lung diseases, asthma
- **I**nfective **D**isease
- **S**eptic shock

Uses of danazol: **EFGHI M P**

Endometriosis
Fibrocystic diseases of breast
Gynecomastia
Hereditary angioneurotic oedema
Infertility
Menorrhagia
Precocious puberty in boys

ORGANOPHOSPHATE POISONING SYMPTOMS

DUMBLES

Diarrhea
Urination
Miosis
Bowel motility increased
Lacrimation
Emesis
Salivation

HYPERGLYCEMIC DRUGS

NOt **FEED H**igh **GLU**cose to **CH**ild **AS** causes **PP** hyperglycemia

Niacin
Ocp
Furosemide
Ethacridine
Encainide
Diazoxide
HIv—protease inhibitor
Growth hormone
GLUcocorticoids

CHlorthalidone
ASparginase
Phenytoin
Pentamidine

ISOTRETINOIN

Side effect—isotretinoin is **CHOTTA drug**
Teratogenic
Cleft palate and facial defects
Hydrocephalus
Outflow obstruction in heart
Thymic hypoplasia
Anotia—stenosis of auditory tube

NITRIC OXIDE DONORS

Highly **PRO** **N**itric **NON**
Hydralazine
PROpofol
Nebivolol
Na nitroprusside
Organic nitrate
Nitrites

LITHIUM USES

LIBRA
Leucopenia
Inappropriate ADH secretion syndrome
Bipolar disorder
Recurrent neuropsychiatric symptoms
Agranulocytosis

THE DRUG CAUSING HIRSUTISM

MAD OCP

- **M**inoxidil
- **A**ndrogens
- **D**iazoxide
- **O**cp contain progesterone
- **C**yclosporins
- **P**henytoin

DRUGS EFFECTIVE IN MRSA

Readymade **S**amsung **LCD TV**

- **R**ifampicin
- **S**treptogramins
- **L**inezolide
- **C**otrimoxazole
- **D**aptomycin
- **T**eicoplanin
- **V**ancomycin

DRUGS USED IN NARCOANALYSIS

Narcoanalysis is a **TEST**

- **T**hiopentone sodium
- **E**thanol
- **S**copolamine
- **T**emazepam

PENICILLIN DOC IN

ACTing **PM PASS L**ist of **T**rains **T**icket

ACTinomycetes
Pneumococci
Meningococcal meningitis
Pasturella
Anthrax
Streptococci
Syphilis
Listeria
Trench fever
Tetanus

PHENYTOIN SIDE EFFECT

PHENYTOIN

P-450 interactions
Hirsutism, **H**yperglycemia
HS—rash, DLE, lymphadenopathy, neutropenia
Enlarged gum
Nystagmus
Yellow browning of skin
Teratogenicity (Fetal hydantoin syndrome)
Osteomalacia
Interference with B_{12} metabolism
megaloblastic anemia
Neuropathies, vertigo, ataxia

SIDE EFFECTS OF CLOZAPINE

MASS

Myocarditis
Agranulocytosis
Seizures
Sialorrhea

USES OF ERYTHROMYCIN AS ALTERNATIVE TO PENICILLIN

STD Gonorrhea

- **S**yphilis
- **T**etanus
- **D**iphtheria
- **G**onorrhea

RITUXIMAB USES

CRAIN

- **C**rohn's disease
- **R**heumatic arthritis
- **A**uto**I**mmune hemolytic anemia
- **N**on-Hodgkin's lymphoma

ACTION OF OPIOID ON μ RECEPTOR

SACRRUM

- **S**edation
- **A**nalgesia
- **C**onstipation
- **R**espiratory depression
- **R**igidity
- e**U**phoria
- **M**iosis

REVERSIBLE ANTICHOLIN ESTERASE

Anti-**R**aging **P**olice **T**ake a **G**reat **DON**

- **A**nticholinesterase
- **R**ivastigmine

Physostigmine
Tacrine
Galantamine
DONepezil

DRUGS CAUSING SLE-LIKE SYNDROME

Plz **C**heck **PCOBOMISHIP**

Procainamide
Chlorpropamide
Barbiturates
OCP
Methyldopa
Interferon-alpha
Sulphonamide
Hydralazine
Isoniazid
Phenytoin

DRUGS THAT ARE ABSORBED IN STOMACH

SNAAP

Sulphonamide
NSAIDs
Aspirin
Alcohol
Phenobarbitone

SUCCINYLCHOLINE FEATURES

SCH

Short surgical procedures
Cause **C**ardiac arrhythmias
Cause **H**yperkalemia

SIDE EFFECTS OF SULPHONAMIDES

SULPHONAMIDES

Stevens-Johnson syndrome
Urticaria
Leucopenia
Photosensitivity
Hemolytic anemia + hepatitis
Obstruction of urinary tract
Nausea
Agranulocytosis
Malaise, **M**egaloblastic anemia
Increased risk of kernicterus in newborn
Depression, **D**rug fever
Eosinophilia
Skin rashes

SYMPATHOMIMETIC HYPERTENSIVES

Many **P**eople **N**ever **M**arry

Mephentermine
Phenylephrine
Noradrenaline
Methoxamine

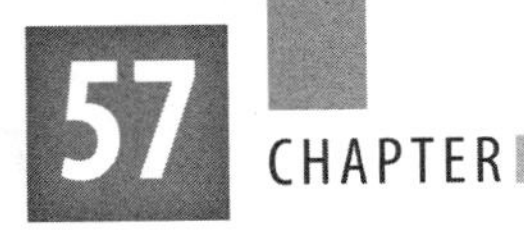

Adverse Effect

Adverse effect	*Drugs causing*
Cleft palate—**PAVAM**	**P**henytoin **A**minopterin **VA**lproate **M**ethotrexate
Alopecia—**GAVA**	**G**entamycin **A**nticancer drug (cisplatin, paclitaxel) **V**alproate **A**nticoagulant (heparin, warfarin)
Cushings syndr**O**me	**C**orticosteroids **O**ral contraceptives
Stevens-Johnson syndrome—**SPPA**	**S**ulphonamide **P**enicillin **P**henytoin **A**llopurinol
Hirsutism—**PCM**	**P**henytoin **C**yclosporin **M**etoclopramide

Contd...

Contd...

Spina **B**ifida	**S**odium valproate Car **B**amazepine
Gingival hypertrophy—CAP	**P**henytoin **A**mlodipine **C**yclosporin
Teeth discoloration—TCI	**T**etracyclin **C**iprofloxacin **I**ron preparations
Oral thrush	Inhalational cortic**O**steroids Antibi**O**tics

58 CHAPTER

Drug of Choice

1. *Malignant hyperthermia:* Dantrolene sodium 1 mg/kg IV
2. *Drug-induced parkinsonism:* Benzhexol 2–20 mg/day
3. *Patent ductus arteriosus:* Indomethacin 0.1–0.2 mg/kg, 12th hourly
4. *Methanol poisoning:* Ethanol loading dose 0.7 mL/kg followed by 0.15 mL/kg/hour drip
5. *Belladonna poisoning:* Physostigmine 0.5 to 2 mg IV
6. *Organophosphorus poisoning:* Atropine 2 mg IV every 10 minute
7. *Motion sickness:* Hyoscine
8. *A/C paracetamol poisoning:* N-acetyl cysteine 150 mg/kg slow IV
9. *BZD overdose:* Flumazenil 0.2 mg IV
10. *Absence seizures:* Sodium valproate, ethosuximide
11. *Myoclonic seizures:* Sodium valproate
12. *A/C schizophrenia:* Haloperidol 2–20 mg/day
13. *A/C morphine poisoning:* Naloxone 0.4–0.8 mg IV every 3 minute
14. *Supraventricular arrhythmia:* Propranolol/verapamil
15. *PSVT:* Adenosine 6–12 mg IM
16. *Typhoid:* Ciprofloxacin 500 mg BD × 10 days
17. *Chancroid:* Cotrimoxazole BD × 7 day/Erythromycin 2 mg/day × 7 days

18. *Pneumocystis carinii:* Cotrimoxazole BD 4–6 times
19. *Syphilis:* Penicillin
20. *Anthrax, actinomycosis, trench fever:* Penicillin G
21. *Rheumatic fever:* Benzathine penicillin 1–2 mg every 4 weeks
22. *Meningitis (pseudomonas):* Ceftazidime + gentamicin
23. *Meningitis (haemophilus influenzae, enterobacteria): Ceftriaxone,* Cefuroxime
24. *Atypical pneumonia:* Tetracycline/erythromycin
25. *Cholera, plague, relapsing fever, rickettsial infection:* Tetracycline
26. *Brucellosis:* Doxycycline 200 mg/day × 6 weeks
27. *Tularemia:* Streptomycin
28. *Pediculosis and scabies:* Permethrin
29. *Neurocysticercosis:* Albendazole
30. *Kala-azar:* Sodium stibogluconate
31. *Dracunculus medinensis:* Metronidazole
32. *Nematode:* Albendazole
33. *Onchocerciasis and strongyloids:* Ivermectin
34. *Whooping cough:* Erythromycin
35. *MRSA:* Vancomycin
36. *Chlamydia trachomatis:* Azithromycin 1 g oral OD
37. *Herpes infection:* Acyclovir
38. *CMV infection:* Ganciclovir/foscarnet
39. *F Malaria:* Chloroquine 600 mg stat followed by 300 mg daily
40. *Cerebral malaria:* Quinine IV
41. *Toxoplasmosis:* Pyrimethamine + sulfadiazine
42. *Trichomonas vaginitis:* Metronidazole 400 mg TDS × 7 days
43. *Amoebic dysentery, giardiasis:* Metronidazole
44. *Pseudomembranous enterocolitis:* Vancomycin/metronidazole

45. *Filariasis:* DEC 2 mg/kg TDS × 2 weeks
46. *Loa loa:* DEC
47. *Tinea infection:* Niclosamide
48. *Hemorrhagic cystitis:* Mesna
49. *Multiple myeloma:* Melphalan
50. *To maintain PDA:* Alprostadil

59 CHAPTER

Treatment of Acute Cases

MYOCARDIAL INFARCTION

- Morphine—analgesic, also decreases anxiety
- Streptokinase as IV infusion within 6 hour for thrombolysis and reperfusion
- Beta-blocker prevent arrhythmia, if arrhythmia present give lignocaine
- ACE inhibitors and ARBS to prevent remolding and subsequent CCF
- *Antiemetic:* H1 blocker (promethazine)
- Oxygenation
- Maintenance of blood volume by slow IV infusion
- For pump failure:
  - Diuretics
  - Vasodilators
  - *Inotropic agents:* Dopamine + dobutamine
- Prevention of thrombus extension by use of aspirin, heparin
- To prevent further attack—**ABC**

  Antiplatelet—aspirin and clopidogrel **(Clolyse:** Clopidogrel 75 mg**)**

  Beta-blocker to prevent reinfarction

  Control hyperlipidemia

HYPERTENSIVE CRISIS

- Sodium nitroprusside 0.25–1.5 μg/kg/min IV infusion in 5% dextrose
- Close monitoring of BP
- *Alternative drugs:* Esmolol, labetalol, hydralazine.

DIABETIC KETOACIDOSIS

- Insulin (loading dose 0.2–0.3 U/kg IV followed by 0.1 U/kg/hour)
- Normal saline to correct dehydration
- 5% glucose to prevent hypoglycemia and cerebral oedema
- Potassium supplementation
- Phosphate
- Antibiotic.

STATUS ASTHMATICUS

- Humidified oxygen inhalation
- Nebulized β_2 adrenergic antagonist (salbutamol 5 mg/terbutaline 10 mg) + anticholinergic agent (ipratropium bromide)
- *Systemic glucocorticoids:* Intravenous hydrocortisone 200 mg IV stat followed by IV hydrocortisone 100 mg 6th hourly or prednisolone 30–60 mg/day depending on the patients condition
- Intravenous fluids to correct dehydration
- *Potassium supplements:* To correct hypokalemia produced by repeated use of salbutamol/terbutaline
- Sodium carbonate to treat acidosis
- Antibiotic to treat infection.

MYXOEDEMA COMA

- Levothyroxine IV/via nasogastric tube
- Inj. Hydrocortisone IV
- Supportive therapy
- Rewarming with blankets
- Ventilatory support correction of electrolyte imbalance.

STATUS EPILEPTICUS

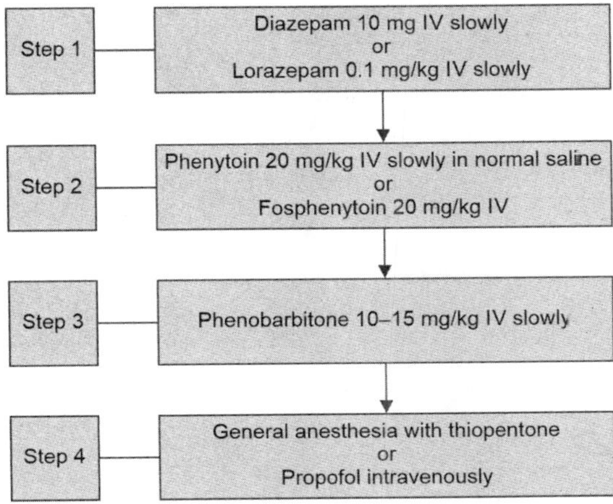

Step 1: Watch for hypotension and respiratory depression
Step 2: Monitor cardiac rhythm and BP
Step 3: Watch for respiratory depression
Step 4: Maintain airway and BP

THYROID STORM

- *Non-selective beta-blocker:* Propranolol 1–2 mg slow IV then 40–80 mg oral 6th hourly
- *Propylthiouracil:* 200–300 mg oral 6th hourly
- *Iopanoic acid:* 0.5–1 g OD oral
- *Corticosteroids:* Hydrocortisone 100 mg IV 8 hourly
- *Diltiazem:* 60–120 mg BD oral

60 CHAPTER

Drug Interaction

Penicillin + tetracycline: Penicillin bactericidal; tetracycline bacteriostatic; efficacy of combination reduced.

Levodopa + metoclopramide: Levodopa relieves parkinsonian symptoms by D2 agonism; metoclopramide blocks central D2 receptors; reduces efficacy of levodopa.

Statins + gemfibrozil: Both causes myopathy and additive toxicity.

Amitriptyline + atropine: Both have anticholinergic action.

Sulfamethoxazole + trimethoprim: Sequential blockade of folate metabolism pathway in microbes.

Amoxicillin + clavulanic acid: Amoxicillin is destroyed by beta-lactamase; clavulanic acid is a beta-lactamase inhibitor; increases amoxicillin concentration.

Nitrate + beta-blockers: Tachycardia caused by nitrate is nullified by beta-blockers action.

Captopril + spironolactone: Dangerous hyperkalemia.

Aspirin + thiazide: Diuretic action of thiazide is PG mediated; aspirin inhibits PG synthesis of diuretic.

OCP + rifampicin: Rifampicin is a microsomal enzyme inducer and increases OCP metabolism and contraceptive failure.

Sucralfate + antacids: Sucralfate polymerises at pH <4; antacid increase pH and prevent action of sucralfate.

Sucralfate + tetracycline/phenytoin: Sucralfate prevents absorption of tetracycline/phenytoin and therapeutic failure.

Diclofenac + salbutamol: NSAID inhibits PG synthesis and arachidonic acid channelled to leukotriene synthesis and bronchoconstriction and worsens asthma.

Astemizole + erythromycin: Erythromycin is a enzyme inhibitor and decreases astemizole metabolism and arrhythmia.

Diuretic + Lithium: Diuretic causes Na^+ loss and decreases Na^+ conc. and lithium gets reabsorbed along with Na^+ and lithium toxicity.

Clopidogrel + warfarin: Clopidogrel—antiplatelet action; warfarin—anticoagulant and increased risk of bleeding.

Frusemide + aminoglycoside: Both are ototoxic drugs and additive toxicity.

Warfarin + ceftriaxone: Hypoprothrombinemia—ADR of ceftriaxone and potentiates the anticoagulant effects of warfarin and increases risk of bleeding.

Neostigmine + atropine: Neostigmine given to reverse muscle paralysis after anesthesia causes muscarinic side effect and reversed by atropine (antimuscarinic).

TCA + clonidine: TCA abolishes antihypertensive action of clonidine by inhibiting its transport into adrenergic neurons.

Cholestyramine + digoxin: Effective blood concentration of digoxin is decreased.

Tolbutamide + salicylate: Salicylate displaces sulfonylureas from PPB sites and cause dangerous hypoglycemia.

Lignocaine + adrenaline: Adrenaline causes vasoconstriction and decreases absorption of lignocaine decreasing the systemic toxicity and increasing the duration of action.

L-dopa + pyridoxine: Pyridoxine as co-factor for carboxylase enzyme and increased peripheral decarboxylation of L-dopa and decreased efficacy.

Ciprofloxacin + theophylline: Ciprofloxacin is a enzyme inhibitor and decreases theophylline metabolism and CVS and CNS toxicity.

Nitrate + CCBs: Nitrate reduces preload (venodilators), CCBs reduces afterload (arteriodilators) and reduces the workload of ischemic heart.

Tetracycline + iron/antacid: Tetracycline absorption decreased and therapeutic failure.

Digoxin + quinidine: Quinidine displaces digoxin from PPB sites and digoxin levels increased (quinidine also decreases the renal clearance of digoxin).

Digoxin + propranolol: Both decreases AV conduction and precipitate AV block.

Penicillin + probenecid: Block tubular secretion of penicillin and decreases penicillin excretion and prolong its duration of action and therapeutic efficacy increased.

Aspirin + methotrexate: Aspirin displaces methotrexate from PPB sites and precipitate methotrexate toxicity.

Index

A

D

E

O

P

Q

R

S

T